Shunts and Problems in Shunts

Monographs in Neural Sciences

Vol. 8

Series Editor
Maynard M. Cohen, Chicago, Ill.

S. Karger · Basel · München · Paris · London · New York · Sydney

Symposium on Shunts and Problems in Shunts, Marseille, June 24–25, 1980

Shunts and Problems in Shunts

Volume Editor
M. Choux, Marseille

79 figures and 42 tables, 1982

S. Karger · Basel · München · Paris · London · New York · Sydney

Monographs in Neural Sciences

National Library of Medicine, Cataloging in Publication

Symposium on Shunts and Problems in Shunts (1980: Marseille, France)
Shunts and problems in shunts: Symposium on Shunts and Problems in Shunts, Marseille, June 24–25, 1980.
Volume editor, M. Choux. – Basel, New York, Karger, 1982.
(Monographs in neural sciences; v. 8)
Preface in French.
1. Cerebrospinal Fluid Shunts – adverse effects – congresses 2. Cerebrospinal Fluid Shunts – congresses 3. Hydrocephalus – surgery – congresses I. Choux, M. (Maurice) II. Title III. Series
ISBN 3–8055–2465–X

Drug Dosage

The authors and the publisher have exerted every effort to ensure that drug selection and dosage set forth in this text are in accord with current recommendations and practice at the time of publication. However, in view of ongoing research, changes in government regulations, and the constant flow of information relating to drug therapy and drug reactions, the reader is urged to check the package insert for each drug for any change in indications and dosage and for added warnings and precautions. This is particularly important when the recommended agent is a new and/or infrequently employed drug.

ISBN 3–8055–2465–X

Contents

Infection in Shunts

Other Complications

Shunt Dependency

Shunt and EEG

Long-Term Results

Technical Problems in Shunts

Shunt Problems Related to the Etiology of Hydrocephalus

Conclusions

Préface

Jacques Rougerie

The foreword has been written by *J. Rougerie,* pioneer in Paediatric Neurosurgery. Our feeling is that it should be kept in its original form.

Ceux qui ont eu, comme moi, la chance de connaître cette étape fantastique qu'a représenté l'avènement des valves, semblent, aujourd'hui, avoir perdu un peu de leur enthousiasme. Il y a d'un côté les optimistes qui évoquent avec une satisfaction très légitime tous ces enfants qui, grâce à la stabilisation durable de leur hydrocéphalie, ont connu une réinsertion sociale parfaite, une scolarité normale sinon brillante. Mais le risque est alors indéniable de considérer le shunt comme un geste mineur et d'en faire une intervention de routine, complètement standardisée. Les pessimistes, dont je suis, ne peuvent oublier la longue série des déboires, des combats difficiles, et souvent malheureux contre les complications, ce qui conduit à un certain degré de découragement.

C'est un peu dans cet état d'esprit que j'ai répondu à l'invitation de *Maurice Choux*. Mais d'emblée j'ai été frappé par la participation qui, toute considération d'amitié mise à part, était importante. Et surtout, à côté de la fine fleur de la neurochirurgie pédiatrique, venue de tous les horizons du monde, il y avait là beaucoup de neurochirurgiens, des jeunes surtout, dont la vocation est loin d'être exclusivement pédiatrique. Manifestement, tous désiraient participer, s'instruire et apporter leur contribution. De fait, dès le début des exposés, on ne pouvait qu'apprécier la sincérité totale avec laquelle chacun s'exprimait, à commencer par les membres des plus grandes équipes internationales.

La matière de ce symposium était d'une richesse extrême mais le Program Committee avait su très judicieusement l'ordonner, autour de passionants exposés, de sorte que chacun pouvait en retirer le maximum d'enseignement:

Nous disposons maintenant de techniques fiables pour identifier les dysfonctionnements des shunts (aigus ou à bas bruit), en préciser le siège et les modalités, donc y apporter (assez aisément dans la plupart des cas) une correction efficace.

Par contre, il est incontestable que l'infection reste le problème majeur et de nombreuses équipes ont défini leur attitude préventive et surtout curative. Je pense personnellement que les efforts faits pour adapter et moduler à chaque cas la technique de *Mac Laurin,* corrélés par des résultats portant sur de longues séries, seront sûrement profitables à tous dans l'avenir.

La tomographie computérisée a eté, en matière d'hydrocéphalie, un apport considérable dans la détection, l'approche anatomique du type de la ou des lésions et la surveillance de l'évolution. Mais il nous a aussi posé de nouveaux problèmes: Que faut-il penser devant un système ventriculaire qui reste globalement ou partiellement dilaté? Quelle interprétation faut-il faire devant la constatation à court ou à long terme de ventricules virtuels? Quelle conduite adopter devant ces épanchements sous-duraux, souvent muets, en fonction de cette délicate notion de 'compliance cérébrale'?

Enfin, j'ai été vivement intéressé par les cas de crânio-sténoses secondaires; non pas, bien sûr, les banales scaphocéphalies mais les formes hypertensives (dont j'ai observé deux cas authentiques) avec les difficultés d'interprétation et de traitement qu'elles comportent.

Je ne puis m'étendre sur le vaste problème que représentent les études minutieuses faites en fonction de l'étiologie, ni sur les réflexions et suggestions techniques, pourtant souvent originales, qui ont été proposées.

Je voudrais terminer sur une réflexion plus générale: ce n'est sûrement pas le fait du hasard si *Maurice Choux* nous a proposé de débuter cette réunion par l'étude des techniques qui permettent d'évaluer aussi exactement que possible le fonctionnement d'un shunt et de la conclure par cette grande question posée par *R. Hemmer* 'Can a shunt be removed?'. Pour en arriver là, nous avons entendu s'affronter, souvent avec passion, des opinions parfois contradictoires sur les possibilités de stabilisation de certaines formes d'hydrocéphalie et sur les critères qui permettraient de l'affirmer. Bien que le mot n'ait pas été prononcé, on sentait planer notre vieux rêve de valve à débit variable, dont je ne désespère pas qu'il devienne un jour réalité.

Je félicite mon ami *Mauric Choux* d'avoir eu le courage de réserver, à la suite du congrès, tout ce qui est acquisition ou prouesse technique pour nous plonger d'emblée dans la réalité de nos problèmes quotidiens. Je voudrais dire aussi à nos collègues plus jeunes qu'ils n'auront pas seulement à 'réviser des shunts', ils auront aussi à réviser bien des idées qui ne représentent qu'une fragile vérité actuelle.

C'est là raison pour laquelle on ne peut dissocier les passionnantes recherches sur la physiopathologie du liquide céphalo-rachidien de nos préoccupations matérielles de tous les jours; le pronostic de l'hydrocéphalie en dépend.

Monogr. neural Sci., vol. 8, pp. 1–6 (Karger, Basel 1982)

Introduction

Maurice Choux

In spite of incessant research and unquestionable advances, the true mechanisms of hydrocephalus remain partially unknown. Advances concerning the physiopathology of hydrocephalus are due to the experimental works carried out in the field of anatomy, physiology and neuroradiology. The fact that some mechanisms of hydrocephalus remain unknown explains the great number of therapeutic procedures.

The treatment of hydrocephalus is one of the richest chapters of the therapeutic field, and the large number of procedures proposed in this field expresses its respective limits and disadvantages. The procedures reducing the secretion of choroid plexuses [*Dandy,* 1918, 1945; *Putnam and Ask-Upmark,* 1934; *Scarff,* 1951, 1970; *Davidoff,* 1948; *Klein,* 1958] did not bring any definitive solution to hydrocephalus In fact, after a temporary stabilization cerebrospinal fluid (CSF) is produced in the same volume and we know now that choroid plexuses are not only CSF structure producers. For the last 60 years a number of intracranial shunt procedures have been performed in cases of ventricular or cisternal obstruction: puncture of the lamina terminalis and of the floor of the third ventricle in the interpeduncular cistern [*Dandy,* 1918, 1945; *Scarff,* 1951, 1970; *Stookey and Scarff,* 1936, *Guiot,* 1973], ventriculo-cisternal shunts [*Torkildsen,* 1947], transcallosal shunts [*Lazorthes,* 1953], ventriculo-subdural shunt [*Forrest et al.,* 1957; *MacNab,* 1966] or third to fourth ventricle shunt [*Dandy,* 1918, 1945; *Leksell,* 1949; *Lapras and Bret,* 1980]. The various intracranial shunts fail because they result in the transformation of obstructive hydrocephalus into communicative hydrocephalus with a possible obstruction of the shunt in most cases. These disappointments have led the physicians to perform new shunting procedures allowing resorption of the CSF. Everything has been tried in this field and CSF has been drained almost everywhere.

Table I. Number of shunts

	Shunts	Atrial shunt	Peritoneal shunt	Ventriculostomy	Others	Shunt now used
Paris (a year)	162	14	148	12		VPS
Nancy	783	506	277	2	20 T	VAS
Toulouse (a year)	50	2	47	1		VPS
Grenoble	247	82	165	13	1 T 1 VP1	VPS
Tours (in 2 years)	119	8	110		1 LP	VPS
Nice (in 4 years)	47	17	29	1		VPS
Algiers	363	48	301	12	2 LP	VPS
Marseilles	940	248	692	22	4 LP	VPS

LP = Lumboperitoneal; VP1 = ventriculopleural; T = Torkildsen.

Among the historic methods we should remember the ureteral shunts [*Matson,* 1949], the mastoid shunts [*Nosik,* 1950], the Fallopian tube shunt [*Harsh,* 1954], the pleural shunts [*Heile,* 1925; *Ransohoff,* 1954], the gallbladder shunts [*Smith et al.,* 1959], to the bowel [*Neumann et al.,* 1959], to the retroperitoneal space [*Aboulker*], to the thoracic duct [*Yokoyana et al.,* 1969], and to the vertebral body [*Radvan-Ziemnowicz,* 1965].

Lumboperitoneal shunts are proposed by some authors in cases of communicative hydrocephalus. In this procedure, a tube is laid from the lumbar spinal subarachnoid space to the peritoneal area [*Jackson and Snodgrass,* 1955; *Picaza,* 1956].

In 1952, *Nulsen and Spitz* found a new approach to the therapy of hydrocephalus. They described a procedure of ventriculo-atrial shunt (CSF was drained into the right auricle of the heart) using a valve. The use of a valve to control the one-way flow of CSF from the lateral ventricle to the heart under relatively constant pressure was a major advance. The shunting of CSF into the blood stream is the artificial doing of a physiological mechanism.

At the end of the last century *Gartner* [1895] and *Payr* [1908] tried to perform vascular shunts but the main difficulty was to avoid the venous counterflow into the ventricular cavities. The introduction of valves prevented this difficulty. The first valves to be used were Holter's and Pudenz's valve. Beside

Table II. Technical procedure and material

	Ventricular cather						Valve			Peritoneal catheter		
	type	reservoir	location	length, cm	control position	CSF pressure	type	pressure	operatory control	type	location	length, cm
Paris	Hol.	yes	occ.	6–7	no	no	Hok.	60–80	no	Hak.	hypoch.	40
Nancy	Hol.	no	par.	6	yes	yes	Hol.	medium	no	Hol.	subcost.	20
	Hak.						Hak.	60–80		Hak.		
Lyon	Hol.	no	occ.	7–8	no	no	Hol.	low pres.	yes	Hol.	hypoch.	20
								medium			midline	
Toulouse	Hak.	yes	fr.	4–6	no	no	Hak.	60–80	no	Hak.	midline	12–20
Grenoble	Hol.	yes	fr.	4–6		no	Hak.	30–40	no	Hak.	subcost.	20
Tours	Hol.	no	occ.	5	no	no	Hol.	medium	yes	Hol.	subcost.	30
Nice	Hol.	no	occ.	6	yes		Hol.	medium	yes	Hol.	subcost.	15
Marseilles	Hol.	yes	occ.	6–7	no	no	Hol.	medium	no	Am.	subcost.	20–25
							Hak.	60–80	no	Am.	subcost.	20–25
Algiers	Hak	no	occ.	8	no	no	Hak.	medium	no	Hak.	hypoch.	18
	Pud.						Pud.	60–80		Pud.		

Hol. = Holter; Hak. = Hakim; Pud. = Pudenz.

Table III. Complications in shunts

	Mechanical: frequency, %	Infection: frequency, %	Subdural effusion: frequency, %
Paris (a year)	18	9.8	1.8
Nancy	20	22 (infant) 8 (adult)	2.5
Toulouse	15	10	2
Grenoble			10
Tours			3
Nice	12	10	
Marseilles	15	8	1.8
Algiers	17	8	5

these two first valves, a number of more or less sophisticated valves were used. The most important are those of: *Ames, Codman, Cordis, and Denver.* But studies are now carried out to simplify technics and material. In this way, some neurosurgeons use a simple catheter inserted into the ventricle and running to the peritoneal cavity with a valve adapted to the distal end of the shunt (Unishunt).

At the appearance of the first valve in 1952 the technic was a ventriculo-atrial shunt. On account of a number of accidents with the cardiac drainage, the ventriculoperitoneal shunt described by *Hausch* [1908], proposed by *Cushing* [1926], and performed by *Cone et al.* [1949] and by *Scott et al.* [1955], was more and more used. Presently 70% of neurosurgeons perform routinely ventriculoperitoneal shunt.

25 years after the insertion of the first shunt with a valve, we thought it was interesting to discuss CSF shunting in the therapy of hydrocephalus and the problems involved in such technics. It was the theme of the symposium which took place in Marseilles at the Hôpital des Enfants de la Timone, during the annual meeting of the International Society for Paediatric Neurosurgery, June 24–25, 1980.

The experimental, physiopathological, etiologic, clinical and radiological considerations and data were purposely left aside. The communications were limited to surgical therapy in hydrocephalus, including technics and complications as well as the follow-up and psycho-intellectual prognosis of a child treated with shunt and valve.

In order to prepare the symposium and to dispose of a sufficient number of statistics in consideration of all the technics used, a questionnaire was sent to the main pediatric neurosurgical centers in France, and in Algeria:

Department of Paediatric Neurosurgery (Prof. *J.F. Hirsch*), Hôpital des Enfants Malades, Paris
Department of Paediatric Neurosurgery (Prof. *Montaut*), Nancy
Department of Neurosurgery (Prof. *C. Lapras*), Hôpital Neurologique, Lyons
Department of Neurosurgery (Prof. *G. Lazorthes*), CHU Purpan, Toulouse
Department of Neurosurgery (Prof. *Barge*), La Tronche, CHU Grenoble
Paediatric Center, Neurosurgery Department (Prof. *J.J. Santini*), Tours
Department of Neurosurgery (Prof. *Duplay, J.L. Roche*), CHU, Nice
Department of Neurosurgery (Prof. *I. Galli*), Hôpital Aid Idir, Alger
Department of Paediatric Neurosurgery (Prof. *M. Choux*), Children's Hospital, La Timone, Marseilles

The answers to this questionnaire are summarized in tables I–III.

References

Cone, W.V.; Lewis, R.D.; Jackson, I.J.: Shunting of cerebrospinal fluid into the peritoneal cavity. Proc. Meet. of American College of Physicians, Montreal 1949.

Cushing, H.: Studies in intracranial physiology and surgery; the third circulation, the hypophysis, the gliomas (Oxford University Press, London 1926).

Dandy, W.E.: Extirpation of the choroid plexus of the lateral ventricles in communicating hydrocephalus. Ann. Surg. *68:* 569 (1918).

Dandy, W.E.: Diagnosis and treatment of strictures of the aqueduct of Sylvius (causing hydrocephalus). Archs Surg., Chicago *51:* 1 (1945).

Davidoff, L.M.: Hydrocephalus and hydrocephalus with meningocele: their treatment by choroid plexectomy. Surg. Clins N. Am. *28:* 416 (1948).

Forrest, D.M.; Laurence, K.M.; MacNab, G.H.: Ventriculo-sub-dural drainage in infantile hydrocephalus. Analysis of early results. Lancet *272:* 1274 (1957).

Guiot, G.: Ventriculo-cisternostomy for stenosis of the aqueduct of Sylvius. Puncture of the floor of the third ventricle with a leucotome under television central. Acta neurochir. *28:* 275–289 (1973).

Harsh, G.R. III: Peritoneal shunt for hydrocephalus utilizing the fimbria of the Fallopian tube for entrance into the peritoneal cavity. J. Neurosurg. *11:* 284 (1954).

Heile, B.: Über neue operative Wege zur Druckentlastung bei angeborenem Hydrocephalus (Ureter-Duraanastomose). Zentbl. Chir. *52:* 2229 (1925).

Jackson, I.J.; Snodgrass, S.R.: Peritoneal shunts in the treatment of hydrocephalus and increased intracranial pressure. A 4-year survey of 62 patients. J. Neurosurg. *12:* 216 (1955).

Klein, M.R.: L'hydrocéphalie du nourrisson (Matson, 1958).

Lapras, C.; Bret, P.: Les sténoses de l'aqueduc de Sylvius. Neuro-Chirurgie *26* (1980).

Lazorthes, G.: La ventriculocisternostomie transcalleuse. Presse méd. *61:* 1210 (1953).

Leksell, L.: A surgical procedure for atresia of the aqueduct of Sylvius. Acta psychiat. neurol. *24:* 559 (1949).

MacNab, G.H.: The development of the knowledge and treatment of hydrocephalus. Devl Med. Child Neurol. *11:* suppl., p. 1 (1966).

Matson, D.D.: A new operation for the treatment of communicating hydrocephalus. Report of a case secondary to generalized meningitis. J. Neurosurg. *6:* 238 (1949).

Neumann, C.G.; Hoen, T.I.; Davis, D.A.: The adaptation of ileoentrectopy to the control of congenital communicating hydrocephalus. Plastic reconstr. Surg. *23:* 159 (1959).

Nosik, W.A.: Ventriculomastoidostomy. Technique and observations. J. Neurosurg. *7:* 236 (1950).

Nulsen, F.E.; Spitz, E.B.: Treatment of hydrocephalus by direct shunt from ventricle to jugular vein. Surg. Forum *2:* 399 (1952).

Payr, E.: Drainage der Hirnventrikel mittelst frei transplantierter Blutgefässe; Bemerkungen über Hydrocephalus. Arch. klin. Chir. *87:* 801–885 (1908).

Picaza, J.A.: The posterior-peritoneal shunt technique for the treatment of internal hydrocephalus in infants. J. neurosurg. *13:* 289 (1956).

Putman, T.J.; Ask-Upmark, E.: The cerebral circulation. XXIX. Microscopic observations on the living choroid plexus and ependyma of the cat. Archs Neurol. Psychiat., *32:* 72 (1934).

Radvan-Ziemnowicz, S.A.: Intravertebral resorption in the treatment of communicating hydrocephalus. Proc. Congr. Chir., Bratislava 1965, p. 27.

Ransohoff, J.: Ventriculo-pleural anastomosis in treatment of midline obstructional neoplasms. J. Neurosurg. *11:* 295 (1954).

Scarff, J.E.: Treatment of obstructive hydrocephalus by puncture of the lamina terminalis and floor of the third ventricle. J. Neurosurg. *8:* 204 (1951).

Scarff, J.E.: The treatment of nonobstructive (communicating) hydrocephalus by endoscopic cauterization of the choroid plexuses. J. Neurosurg. *33:* 1 (1970).

Scott, M.; Wycis, H.T.; Murtagh, F.; Reyes, V.: Observations on ventricular and lumbar subarachnoid peritoneal shunts in hydrocephalus in infants. J. Neurosurg. *12:* 165 (1955).

Smith, G.W., Moretz, W.H.; Pritchard, W.L.: Ventriculo-biliary shunt. A new treatment for hydrocephalus. Surg. Forum *9:* 701 (1959).

Stookey, B., Scarff, J.: Occlusion of the aqueduct of Sylvius by neoplastic and non-neoplastic processes with a rational surgical treatment for relief of the resultant obstructive hydrocephalus. Bull. Neurol. Inst. N.Y. *5:* 348 (1936).

Torkildsen, A.: Ventriculocisternostomy. A palliative operation in different types of noncommunicating hydrocephalus (Johan Grundt Tanum Forlag, Oslo 1947).

Yokoyana, I.; Aoki, H.; Tatebayashi, K.; Hirai, T.; Matsumoto, T.; Fukushima, T.: Ventriculolymphangiostomy. A shunting operation for hydrocephalus to drain cerebrospinal fluid into the thoracic duct. Folia psychiat. neurol. jap. *13:* 305 (1959).

Prof. M. Choux, Hôpital des Enfants, La Timone, Rue Saint-Pierre
F–13005 Marseille (France)

Monogr. neural Sci., vol. 8, pp. 7–11 (Karger, Basel 1982)

A Survey of Complications, Their Avoidance and Results in Ventriculo-Atrial Shunts from 1961 to 1978

R. Hemmer

Neurosurgical Department of the University of Freiburg, FRG

Over two decades after the pioneer work of *Spitz-Holter* and *Pudenz-Heyer,* the treatment of hydrocephalus has reached a point where a critical assessment of methods, complications, and late results seems useful. I do not wish to enter into the discussion of numerous modifications of the drainage systems. It is certain that hitherto none of the used systems and details are able to exclude complications. None of the systems resists in long-term follow up the biological demands. Growth processes, obstructions of the catheter, aging of the material, etc. will in due course take place in all shunts implanted in babies.

Some complications are avoidable or reducible. Three of these we pointed out in 1967 and 1969 [3–5]. Of primary importance are *dislocations of the catheters.* Our studies from 1961 to 1971 [2] have shown that 27% of the complications were dislocations of the ventricular or the heart catheter. After suggesting an innovation for the Holter system and the introduction of simple silicone sleeves with application of a metal bulge to the metallic ends in 1967 and 1968 this complication could be reduced within 4 years from 16 to 1% in ventricular catheters and from 11 to 0% in heart catheters. The total amount of slipping catheters from 1961 to 1976 was reduced to 16%. We suggested a similar innovation for the Pudenz system a few years later.

Another complication is due to the *localization* of the *ventricular catheter.* Blood, brain tissue, but especially choroid plexus may penetrate into the ventricular catheter and the valve. In the past several specially constructed ventricular catheters have been manufactured. However, a mere change of shape alone cannot prevent the obstruction. The best we can do is to place the catheter into the anterior horn, where there is very little plexus.

A further complication concerns the valve itself [6, 11]; this we denoted in 1969 as *relative valve insufficiency.* Either the amount of CSF to be drained is greater than the capacity of the valve, or the capacity of the valve is too large. The checking of the valve during operation should not be limited by forcing water through the valve. The check must include exact flow characteristics. We use a hydrostatic glass manometer filled with 0.9% saline for checking the flow characteristics in drops per minute down to 100 mm H_2O. In a similar way, we proceed with our follow-up patients in the outpatient department.

To a certain extent the formation of a *thrombosis* may be influenced. We know that thrombosis hardly is seen if the catheter is localized within the auricle of the heart. The early preventive reimplantation of the heart catheter in the clinically healthy can avoid thrombosis. The risk of thrombosis corresponds to the amount of displacement of the distal catheter in cranial direction and the duration of the displacement. This was clearly shown intraoperatively when performing preventive lengthening of the catheter – first suggested by *Tsingoglou and Forrest* [12]. We found intraoperatively that thrombosis occurred after indwelling catheters were left in situ for 2 years in 20%, up to 6 years in 67%, and up to 14 years in 85%. In 100 patients with preventive reimplantation of the heart catheter we found the end of the catheter 59 times within the jugular vein, 35 times within v. brachiocephalica and in 6 within v. cava superior. In 37 patients we needed a peritoneal drainage. The shunt could be removed in 4 patients. One fact seems very important to us: in 37% of children who seemed to be in good health we found an increased intraventricular pressure of 100–480 mm H_2O. [1].

Sepsis is even a graver risk. Though it occurred in only 5% in our last investigation in 1976, it was lethal in one third of the cases. The use at operation of newer aseptic solutions, covering of the skin with plastic foil, perioperative Co-trim preparations (Bactrim, Eusaprim) seems to be effective. Repeated revisions increase the incidence of infections. When infections occur the shunt must usually be removed before they can be brought under control.

Our analysis of *mortality* is based on autopsy findings (41%) and clinical data between 1961 and 1978 [9]. There were 590 children with hydrocephalus excluding hydrocephalus caused by tumors. The total mortality to date amounted to 137 (23%), the operative mortality to 0.6%. Neonates accounted for 52% of the deaths, infants for 31%. Children over 6 years of age accounted for only 17–18% of the deaths.

Statistical evaluation showed in 1961–1973 that the life expectancy after 5 years of age was 96% (P_{05} = 0.955) for hydrocephalus communicans, 83% (P_{05} = 0.828) for hydrocephalus with myelocele, and 78% (P_{05} = 0.779) for obstructive hydrocephalus [7, 8]. The probable mortality up to the age of 10 is seen in figure 1. Mortality amounted for 29% in children who were operated on 16–18 years ago, and to 41 and 47% in children who were operated on 14 and 15 years ago. The sharp drop in the mortality from 1966/67 onward is particularly striking. This is not so much due to new operative technical changes, but rather to a more intensive follow-up of the children and better informed parents. The continued co-work between surgeon, pediatrician and parents is a prerequisite for successful care.

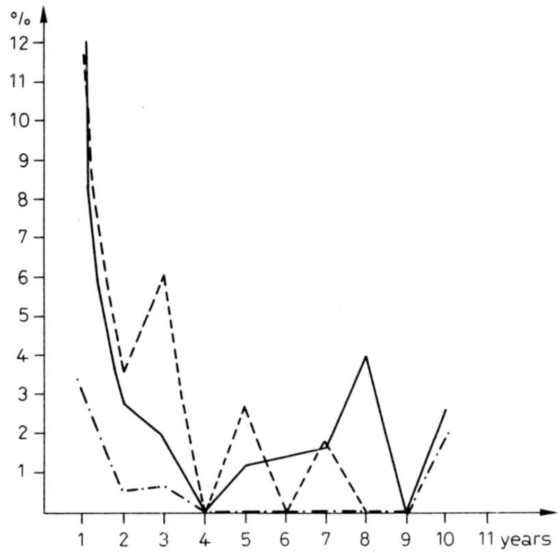

Fig. 1. Statistic likelihood of mortality for 10 years. ——— = Myelocele; – – – = hydrocephalus occlusus; ·——— · = hydrocephalus communicans.

The results relating to the *mental development* underline the importance of early operation. Impressively we can see this in myeloceles, who were from the beginning of their life in medical aftercare. Since 1970 we performed in our outpatient department 605 psychological tests (with the support of Deutsche Forschungsgemeinschaft), and could confirm our first results. The mental development is significantly higher in children with myeloceles than in the other group of hydrocephalus. Longitudinally we saw in 62% of the tested children the same intelligence quotient, in 24% better results, and in 14% worse results. The better results are mostly based upon the stability of the psychical conditions, a greater ability to work, and a harmonized maturity. The causes of decrease of intellectual ability lie partly in the progression of cerebral damage, convulsions, etc.

The school situation is marked by the high percentage of schoolable myeloceles (99%), in contrast to the ability to attend school in 77% of other hydrocephalic infants. If we consider the group of teenagers which was operated on 14–18 years ago, there lies the interesting question: What happens in relation to their apprenticeship? We found out that in the survival group of 108 registered teenagers (28 myeloceles, 80 hydrocephalus communicans and occlusus) 25 enter an apprenticeship, 6 an occupation training year and, from a subgroup of 26, 13 enter secondary school, 6 technical school, and 7 grammar school. We estimate that 53% of these teenagers will practice an occupation. This can be a commercial

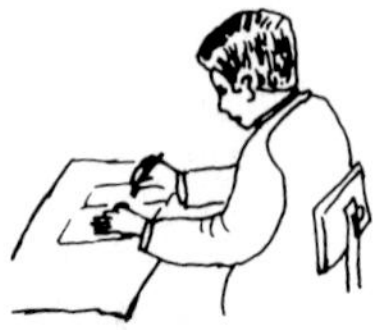	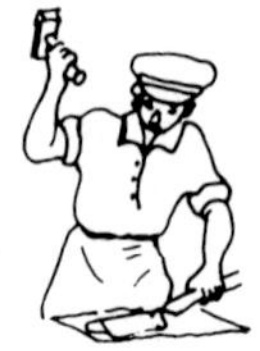	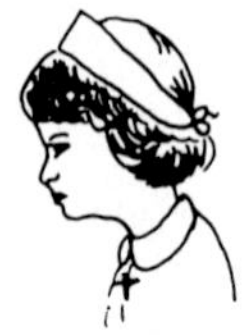	
Commercial employments (10)	Craftsmanship (9)	Social worker (6)	Higher education (6)
Salesman (1) Office worker (2) Office mechanic (1) Bank clerk (1) Civil service (1) Postman (1) Business administration (1) Commercial school teaching (1) Technical draftsman (1)	Shoemaker (1) Mason (1) Mechanic (1) Gardener (3) Stock-keeper (1) Tailoress (1) Farming (1)	Geriatric nurse (1) Infant nurse (1) Kindergarten (1) Nursing (1) Housekeeping (1) Domestic science Teaching (1)	

Fig. 2. Ages 15–18 in apprenticeship and higher education.

one, handicraft or an occupation of social worker (fig. 2). It may happen that some of the patients attending grammar school choose an academic occupation. 28% of the children are in a special school for physically and mentally handicapped, including 9 children in protected workshops. The rest of 10% are children put out to be nursed.

One word on the very severe group of myeloceles. We know from our continued research in mental development that this group has on average a higher mental development and, despite the physical handicap of being chairbound and incontinent, many of this group are fulltime employed. *Laurence and Beresford* [10] found that 70% of the non-operated myeloceles – this is a selected group – are in such a situation.

References

1 Böhm, B.; Hemmer, R.: Die Bedeutung der präventiven Neuanlage des Herzkatheters bei operierten Hydrocephalus-Kindern. Mschr. Kinderheilk. *127:* 357–359 (1979).

2 Busse, G.: Komplikationen mit der Hirnseitenventrikel-Herzohrdrainage bei 586 Patienten mit Hydrocephalus; Diss. Med., Freiburg i.Br. (1974).

3 Hemmer, R.: Complications relating to ventricular-venous shunts: a five-year study. Devl. Med. Child Neur. *13:* 108–112 (1967).

4 Hemmer, R.: Komplikationen beim atrio-ventrikulären Shunt und ihre Vermeidung. Z. Kinderchir. *5:* 10–24 (1967).
5 Hemmer, R.: Dringliche chirurgische Eingriffe an Gehirn, Rückenmark und Schädel im frühen Säuglingsalter (Enke, Stuttgart 1969).
6 Hemmer, R., Potthoff, P.C.: Die Ventilinsuffizienz bei ventriculo-auriculären Drainagen. Z.Kinderchir. *8:* 11–16 (1970).
7 Hemmer, R.: Surgical treatment of hydrocephalus: complications, mortality, developmental prospects. Z.Kinderchir. *22:* 443–452 (1977).
8 Hemmer, R.; Czink, A.: Lethality of children with hydrocephalus and ventriculo-atrial shunts. Z.Kinderchir. *21:* 313–326 (1977).
9 Hemmer, R.: Therapie des Hydrocephalus. Mschr. Kinderheilk. *127:* 337–341 (1979).
10 Laurence, K.M.; Beresford, A.: Degree of physical handicap, education and occupation of 51 adults with spina bifida. Br. J. prevent. soc. Med. *30:* 197–202 (1976).
11 Potthoff, P.C.; Hemmer, R.: Valve insufficiency in ventriculo-atrial shunts. Devl. Med. Child Neur. *20:* 38–41 (1969).
12 Tsingoglou, S.; Forrest, D.M.: Therapeutic and prophylactic lengthening of distal catheter of the Holter ventriculo-atrial shunt. Devl. Med. Child Neur. *16:* suppl., p. 35 (1968).

Prof. Dr. R. Hemmer, Neurosurgical Clinic of the University, Hugstetter Strasse 55, D–7800 Freiburg (FRG)

Monogr. neural Sci., vol. 8, pp. 12–15 (Karger, Basel 1982)

Shunts and Shunt Problems

Luciano Basauri, Arturo Zuleta
Neurosurgical Institute, Santiago, Chile

In the 20-year period 1959–1979, more than 1,000 internal shunt valve systems for the treatment of hydrocephalus of infants and adults were inserted in our institute. Of them, 500 cases under 15 years of age were selected for the present presentation.

Material (table I)

Type of Hydrocephalus (fig. 1)

95% of the series corresponded to *non-tumoral hydrocephalus:* only 5% were due to a tumor of the CNS. *Obstructive hydrocephalus* constituted 98% of the group, being 44% of the cases secondary to an intraventricular obstruction, the most frequent aqueductal stenosis (85% of the group). *Extraventricular obstruction* was the cause in 52% of the patients. Pyogenic meningitis, congenital hydrocephalus and birth trauma were the most frequent pathologies (62% of the group). In only 7 cases it was possible to assume overproduction of CSF as the cause of hydrocephalus.

Methods of Study

Before 1968 the patients were handled with subdural taps, X-rays of the skull, PEG and/or PVG and carotid angiography (as an exception). The use of gammacisternography and/or gammaventriculography for evaluation of the CSF circulation pattern and the functional status of the shunts were introduced in 1968. CT scan is available since 1978.

Table I. Hydrocephalus[1] – Neurosurgical Institute, Santiago-Chile: 1959–1979

< 6 months	< 1 year	1–5 years	6–10 years	11–15 years
299 cases 60%	382 cases 76%	62 cases	28 cases	28 cases

[1] From more than 1,000 cases of children and adult hydrocephalus 500 patients were selected: 288 males (57.6%); 212 females (42.4%).

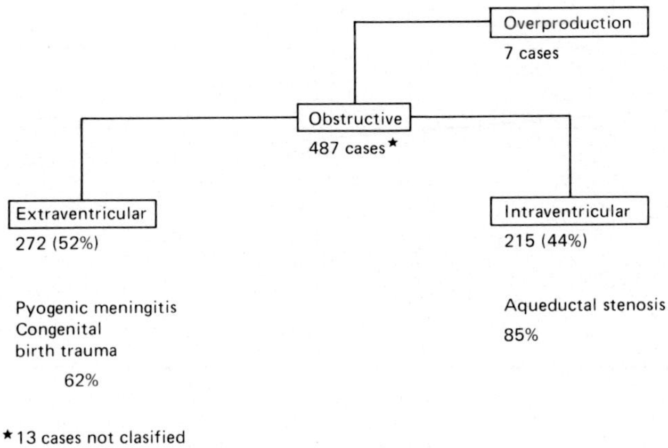

Fig. 1. Classification of hydrocephalus.

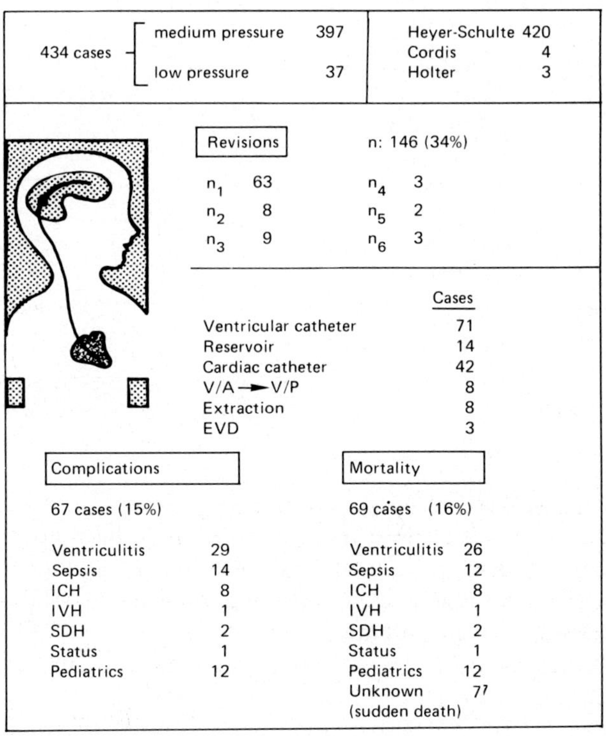

Fig. 2. V/A shunts.

Table II. V/P shunts

Complications 34 cases (55%)			Mortality 23 cases (38%)	
	wound	4	Sepsis	5
Infection 24	sepsis	3	Ventriculitis	13
	ventriculitis	17	SDH	2
			Salicylic intoxication	1
Skin necrosis		5	Sudden death	2
Fistula		3		
SDH		2		
L/P shunts		5		

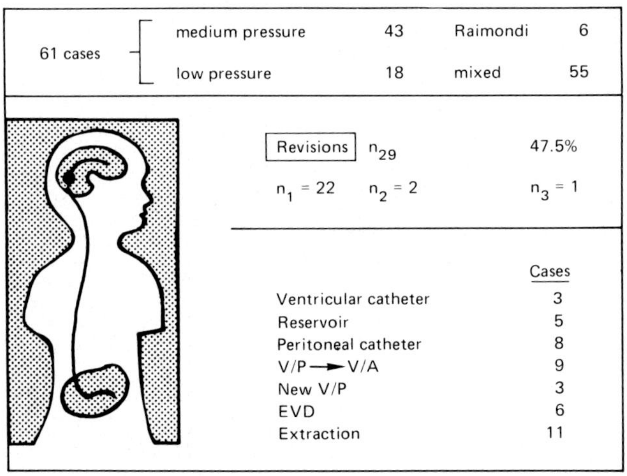

Fig. 3. V/P shunts.

Results

Ventriculo-Atrial Shunts (V/A Shunts): 434 cases (fig. 2)

Revisions. 146 cases – 34 %. The most frequent location of the failures were the ventricular catheter, cardiac catheter and the reservoir. In 8 cases it was necessary to remove the prosthesis and in 3 patients an external ventricular drainage was employed as a transient solution.

Complications. 76 cases – 15%. The most frequent were ventriculitis, sepsis and pediatric complications.

Mortality. 69 cases – 16%. In 60% of the cases the causes of death were ventriculitis and/or sepsis.

Ventriculo-Peritoneal Shunt (V/P Shunts): 61 cases (table II, fig. 3)

Revisions. 29 cases – 47.5%. The most frequent causes of failure were obstruction of the catheters and the reservoir. In 9 children the V/P shunt was replaced with a V/A shunt. In another 3 a new V/P shunt was inserted. 6 cases were submitted to transient external ventricular drainage.

Complications. 34 cases – 55%. The most frequent infection in 24 patients.

Mortality. 23 cases – 38%. 78% of the group died after an infection (sepsis or ventriculitis).

Remarks

In the authors' opinion and despite the appearance of CT scanners, the functional evaluation of CSF circulation with radioisotopes and the monitoring of ventricular CSF pressure with estimation of the compliance and CSF production are important parameters for the therapeutic decision in a group of patients with normal or low-pressure hydrocephalus (the so-called arrested or compensated hydrocephalus). The methods are also useful for the investigation of shunt malfunction. Infection is 'the' problem of shunt morbidity and mortality. The cleaning and protection of the skin during the procedure and the use of i.v. intraoperative antibiotics are necessary to avoid or decrease such complications.

In the present material most of the patients were of the low-income population. Premature, undernourished and low weight patients were common. Skin necrosis (and subsequent infection) are more frequent in that kind of patient. The use of reservoir (of any kind) must be eliminated in such cases. The V/P shunt had a higher morbidity and mortality as well as a higher number of revisions. Some of the aspects already analyzed seem to account for this apparent failure. Shunt valves are not a good treatment for hydrocephalus, but are the best we have for the time being. Whenever possible the insertion of a shunt valve must be avoided. The earth is composed of different worlds, so its is impossible and unwise to extrapolate results between rich countries and the third world.

L. Basauri, MD, Neurosurgical Institute, B.O. Box 3717, Santiago (Chile)

Monogr. neural Sci., vol. 8, pp. 16–17 (Karger, Basel 1982)

Late Postoperative Results in Hydrocephalia of the Infant

A. V. Ciurea

The Neurosurgery Clinic of Bucharest, 'Dr. G. Marinescu' Hospital
(Director: Prof. Dr. *C. Arseni*), Bucharest, Romania

Between 1963 and 1978 a total of 464 cases of hydrocephalia in infants were operated in the Neurosurgery Clinic of Bucharest. In none of the cases was there an expanding intracranial process. The technique applied in all the cases consisted in ventriculo-cardiac drainage with the Holter valve. The type of valve that was chosen depended on the intraventricular pressure, and this was directly evaluated during surgery. The intraoperative death rate in our patients was nil. In the course of the immediate postoperative period a total of 17 patients (3.66%) died, and another 20 patients (4.31%) died in the later postoperative stages. Thus, the death rate of the entire group was of 7.97% (37 cases). We should also mention the fact that 48 of the patients did not come back for control, representing 10.34% of the total.

On the other hand 379 of the cases (81.68%) could be followed in the later stages for periods between 1 and 15 years, and these were classified, according to clinical examination, to neurological, ophthalmologic, psychologic, pediatric, and other criteria, in three groups. Thus, we found good and very good results in 93 patients (24.53%), moderately good results in another 210 patients (55.40%), and poor results in 76 patients (20.05%). It is certain that the results obtained were less influenced by the valve type, by the surgical method used, or by the drainage technique than by the surgical indication of hydrocephalia.

Postoperative complications were noted in only 98 patients (25.85%). Infectious complications occurred in 27 cases (7.12%) and mechanical complications in 71 (18.73%). In the 71 patients with mechanical complications, 124 checks of the draining tubing were made. In 47 patients a single check was necessary, while in the others between two and five checks had to be made.

The most frequent mechanical complications were recorded in the ventricular cathether. The longer the period of follow-up the more numerous were the complications. In view of reducing the incidence of the complications a strict program was applied, aimed at avoiding cranio-cerebral trauma, infections, immunoprophylaxis, exposure to sun, and physical efforts in the first 5 years after the operation. The patients were repeatedly hospitalized in the Neurosurgery Clinic of Bucharest upon the development of the first signs of failure, and corticoid therapy was immediately administered, under antibiotic protection. Drainage tubing was checked only in case where mechanical obstruction was certain.

In none of the cases did we have to apply ventriculo-peritoneal drainage, because of the multiple mechanical complications of the obstructive type encountered described in connection with this surgical procedure.

A.V. Ciurea, MD, The Neurosurgery Clinic of Bucharest, 'Dr. G. Marinescu' Hospital, Bucharest (Romania)

Monogr. neural Sci., vol. 8, pp. 18–20 (Karger, Basel 1982)

Statistical Assessment of Hydrocephalus Operations Performed on 125 Children

J.C. Suárez, Z.M. Sfaello, R. Castillo Morales, P. Saladino, M.A. Echegaray
Department of Neurosurgery, Children's Hospital, Cordoba, Argentina

We are here analyzing the case of 125 hydrocephalic children whose ages, when admitted, ranged between 1 month and over 6 years. 81.6% of the sample, however, corresponded to children of under 8 months of age. There were 74 boys and 51 girls in this sample. There was no parental consanguinity in any of the patients in the sample, but there were family precedents of the same type of malformation in 5 of these cases, and of various other developmental anomalies in another 7. It was found that, in 11 cases, parents had had problems to conceive, and that some of them had been treated, whereas others had not. Signs of prenatal pathologies, which had included biological, physical and chemical factors, were also observed in another 25 children in the sample. Cases where the hydrocephalus corresponded to stenosis of the Sylvian aqueduct, to complex malformation of the encephalus and to cortical subarachnoid cysts, were frequently observed in both pathological births and others which required cesarean operation.

The etiology for these 125 cases of hydrocephalus was as follows: congenital in 89 cases, post meningitis in 25, post hemorrhages in 6, and by tumors in 5. The congenital etiology corresponded as follows: stenosis of Sylvian aqueduct in 47 cases, congenital communicant in 17, Arnold-Chiari's malformation in 14, complex malformation of encephalus in 8, congenital closure of the fourth ventricle outlets in 3. The hemorrhage etiology was as follows: dystocic birth in 3 cases, head injuries in 2, rupture of angioma in 1, and finally the tumor etiology was due to craniopharyngioma in 2 cases, papilloma of the choroid plexus in 1, adenocarcinoma of the choroid plexus in 1, and in another case it was due to a tumor of the brain stem.

There were 46 patients suffering from congenital anomalies of the central nervous system, conditions associated to hydrocephalus, 43 of which were lumbosacral myelomeningoceles and occipital encephaloceles in another 3. The diagnostic procedures employed for this sample were the following: 182 neuroradiological studies, 30 electroencephalograms and 2 isotope cisternograms. The latter were performed on children suffering from normal pressure communicant hydrocephalus. As for the electroencephalograms, they were normal in 5 cases and abnormal in the other 25, out of which 21 were abnormally diffuse and the other 4 focalized.

The neuroradiological studies comprised 87 pneumoventriculographs, 76 pneumoencephalographs, 9 computer tomographs, 7 carotid arteriographs and 3 vertebral arteriographs. The cortical mantle was under 11 mm in 26 patients, between 11 and 20 mm in 68, between 21 and 30 mm in 23 and over 30 mm in 8 children. Its thickness was observed in patients with hydrocephalus caused by intracranial tumors, by secondary hemorrhage following head injuries, by rupture of angioma and by papilloma of the choroid plexus.

The treatment for the hydrocephalus in the children in this sample was surgical, medical in convulsive children, and rehabilitation. The latter was applied in only 71 patients, and early stimulation (Bobath and motor-point techniques) was employed. Anti-convulsive drugs were prescribed for 85 children, some of whom exhibited either the West or Lennox syndrome. The surgical treatment consisted of shunts applied in 124 cases, resection of tumors in 4 and, in the remaining cases, section of the tentorium, resection of left frontotemporal angioma and suboccipital craniectomy. The resection of tumors corresponded as follows: craniopharyngioma in 2 cases, papilloma of the choroid plexus in 1 and in another adenocarcinoma of the choroid plexus. The extracranial derivations employed included ventriculoatrial shunt in 63 cases and ventriculoperitoneal shunt in 61 cases. The valves used in this series were of the following types: Pudenz in 91 cases, Medix in 25, Holter in 5 and Mayo in 3. 78 valve revisions were performed, out of which 51 were being made for the first time, 16 for the third and 3 for the fourth time. The catheters most frequently revised were the ventricular in 24 cases, the peritoneal in 16 and the venous cathether in 12; there were 15 valve replacements and, in the 11 remaining cases, combined revisions of the various cathethers were made.

Surgical complications were observed in 16 patients; in 12 cases they were due to infection, CSF fistulas in 3 cases and in 1 case there was a scar in the scalp. These 16 complications represented 12.8% of all the patients and 7.6% of all the operations performed which totaled 209 and included derivative operations, valve revisions, etiological and physiological operations, such as suboccipital decompression and section of the tentorium. May we point out that the patient on whom the latter techniques were applied was the only one not requiring a valve.

Out of the 125 patients in the sample, 88 survived the operation up to 9 years and 37 died. General mortality was 29.6% and surgical mortality 7.6%. Death was due to surgical causes in 16 cases, by infections not involving the CNS in 12, by uncorrected valve dysfunction in 6, by tumors in 2 cases and by renal insufficiency in 1 case. Of the 16 deaths which had surgical causes, 9 were due to infection, 3 to injury of the brain stem and, in the remaining 4 cases, it was caused by hydropericardium, lung embolism and pneumothorax. In 1 case, the injury of the brain stem corresponded to exclusion of a fourth ventricle, in another to bilateral neurinoma of the accoustic nerve and, in the third case, to an operated valvular dysfunction, observed in a girl who was decerebrated on admission.

Assessment of morbidity in the 88 patients who survived was based on the following: psychointellectual development, motility, and sphincterial functions. Psychointellectual development has been normal in 43 of these children and abnormal in the other 45, in whom psychomotor retardation was observed. This retardation is mild in 6 children, moderate in 18 and serious in 21. Mortility is normal in 50 patients and abnormal in 38; 21 of these, having been operated on for lumbosacral myelomeningoceles, show motor deficiencies in their lower limbs; 9 show lower limb spasticity; 6 present hemiparesis and 2 monoparesis. Of the 21 children with lower limb motor deficiencies on account of their myelomeningoceles, 13 have paraparesis and 8 have paraplegia.

The urinary sphincter is normal in 65 patients and abnormal in 23 patients who show various degrees of neurogenic bladder on account of their myelomeningoceles. In 69 cases, the anal sphincter is normal and abnormal in 19 patients on account of spina bifida. In only 15 out of 23 children showing dysfunction of the vesical sphincter was a sphincter electromyogram taken, which showed various degrees of injury.

Conclusion

We have presented 125 children with hydrocephalus of different etiologies who were given comprehensive treatment by a team of specialists and whose general and surgical mortality was 29.6 and 7.6% respectively. The psychointellectual development has been normal in 50% of the 88 surviving patients and their school performance is good; another 27% attend differential schools, and their performance is also good, with good future prospects of their achieving autonomous behavior.

J.C. Suárez, MD, Department of Neurosurgery, Children's Hospital, Cordoba (Argentina)

Monogr. neural Sci., vol. 8, pp. 21–25 (Karger, Basel 1982)

Management of Hydrocephalus

Harold J. Hoffman, E. Bruce Hendrick, Robin P. Humphreys
Division of Neurosurgery, University of Toronto; Hospital for Sick Children, Toronto, Canada

Introduction

All patients admitted to the neurosurgical service at the Hospital for Sick Children, Toronto, have relevant data in regard to their disease as well as their operative management, placed on protocol sheets which are then key punched into the University of Toronto computer. This has been carried out on a prospective basis on all patients admitted to our service for the past 7 years and on a retrospective basis on all patients with brain tumor and hydrocephalus managed in our institution dating back to 1950.

The present data include all patients with hydrocephalus who were treated at our institution during the years 1960–1980. We have excluded patients who were shunted elsewhere in any part of their history, patients who have been lost to follow-up within 2 years of treatment, patients who have significant missing data in their files and patients with less than 6 months follow-up.

Material

During the years 1960–1980, 1,477 patients were treated for hydrocephalus at our institution. 957 patients (64.8%) had a VP shunt as their initial form of management for their hydrocephalus, 192 patients (13.0%) had a VA shunt as their initial form of management, and 328 patients (22.2%) had an LP shunt as their initial form of management. The subsequent review is based on the type of shunt used initially and does not reflect the child's present shunt, if the original shunt was converted to some other type. In the case of infected shunts, however, the data will reflect the actual infected shunt, rather than the child's original shunt.

Our management changed over the years. Table I indicates very vividly the decreasing popularity of the VA shunt in our institution, consistent with the trend seen in many institutions throughout the world.

Table I.

Year of shunting	Type of initial shunt			
	VP	VA	LP	total
1960–1964	41	60	73	174
1965–1969	173	84	92	349
1970–1974	369	30	102	501
1975–1979	374	18	61	453
Total	957	192	328	1,477

Table II. Shunt survival time: blockage within 6 months of insertion

	VP (%)	VA (%)	LP (%)	Total (%)
1960–1964	30/41 (73.1)	27/60 (45)	28/73 (38.3)	85/174 (48.8)
1965–1969	119/173 (68.7)	30/84 (35.7)	28/92 (30.4)	177/526 (33.6)
1970–1974	164/369 (44.4)	12/30 (40)	33/102 (32.3)	209/501 (41.7)
1975–1979	128/374 (34.2)	4/18 (22)	14/61 (22.9)	146/453 (32.2)
Total	441/957 (46)	73/192 (38.0)	103/192 (53.6)	617/1,654 (37.3)

Pathogenesis of the Hydrocephalus

Myelodysplasia was the commonest condition for which hydrocephalus was treated in our institution. Of the 1,477 patients treated, 430 (29.1%) had myelodysplasia. A further 278 (18.8%) had tumor as the cause of their hydrocephalus, 157 (10.6%) had a post-traumatic hydrocephalus, 84 (5.7%) had post-infectious hydrocephalus, 167 (11.3%) had congenital adueduct stenosis, and 41 (2.8%) had the Dandy-Walker syndrome.

Shunt Survival Time (table II)

During the early years VP shunts tended to block very quickly after insertion. This was no doubt due to the short lengths of tubing then used and the type of material used. During 1960–1964, 73.1% of VP shunts blocked within the first 6 months of insertion. The situation improved as a result of the use of better material and better techniques as demonstrated by the fact that of VP shunts inserted during 1975 to 1979, only 34.2% blocked within 6 months of insertion. VA shunts tended to survive for longer periods of time without blockage than VP shunts. During 1960–1964, 45% blocked within 6 months of insertion whereas during 1975–1979, 22% blocked within the first 6 months. LP shunts had the longest survival time of all with only 38.3% blocking within the first 6 months of insertion during 1960–1964 and 22.9% blocking within 6 months during 1975–1979.

Subsequent Procedures (table III)

Shunt obstruction, shunt infection, and shunt migration are common complications which of necessity lead to further operative procedures for the treated hydrocephalic patient. We looked at our results on the basis of 5-year periods from 1960 to 1980. We

Table III. Subsequent procedures

Time	Procedures per patient (%)			
	VP	VA	LP	total
1960–1964	172/41 (4.2)	187/60 (3.1)	265/73 (3.6)	624/174 (3.6)
1965–1969	719/173 (4.1)	223/84 (2.6)	346/92 (3.8)	1.288/349 (3.7)
1970–1974	1,193/369 (3.2)	91/30 (3.0)	334/102 (3.3)	1,618/501 (3.2)
1975	134/62 (2.2)	10/3 (3.3)	28/12 (2.3)	172/77 (2.2)
Total	2,218/645 (3.6)	511/177 (2.8)	973/279 (3.5)	3,702/1,101 (3.4)

found that with the passage of time and the improvement of techniques and the increasing experience in the management of hydrocephalus the number of procedures carried out per patient decreased significantly. During the 5-year period between 1960 and 1964 there were 41 patients treated with VP shunt and these patients had 172 operative procedures in the 5 years after their initial insertion, indicating 4.2 procedures per patient over 5 years. Of the 62 patients who had a VP shunt inserted in the year 1975 there have been 134 operative procedures in the 5 years since 1975 indicating a procedure rate of 2.2 procedures per patient in 5 years. Similar trends were seen with LP shunts and to a lesser extent with VA shunts.

Results

Of the 1,477 patients with hydrocephalus managed in our institution during this period, 279 (18.9%) have died. 176 of these patients died of their primary disease which was usually a brain tumor. A further 86 died of shunt malfunction and 17 died of sundry other causes.

Arachnoiditis

During the early years, all of our lumboperitoneal shunts were made of polyethylene. 73 of these were inserted during 1960–1964 and a further 92 between 1965 and 1969. During 1973 we began using silastic T-tubes so that during the era of 1970–1974, 57 polyethylene tubes were inserted as compared to 46 silastic tubes. During the years 1975–1979, 10 polyethylene tubes were inserted compared to 50 silastic T-tubles. Of the 232 polyethylene shunts that have been used in our institution, 47 patients have evidence of arachnoiditis with 24 of these having a major neurologic deficit resulting from the arachnoiditis. Of the 92 silastic shunts inserted, we have had 4 patients with arachnoiditis with only 1 of these having a major neurologic deficit as a result of the arachnoiditis.

Table IV. Frequency of organism in infected shunt

	Myelodys-plasia	Other non-comm. hydro.	Neo-plasm	Comm. hydro.	Total (%) n = 317
Staphylococcus epidermidis	56	38	7	21	122 (38.5)
Staphylococcus aureus	23	14	4	16	24 (17.9)
E. coli	10	7	3	4	24 (7.5)
Streptococcus	9	6	0	1	16 (5.0)
Pseudomonas	7	2	0	0	9 (2.8)
Proteus	6	3	0	0	9 (2.8)
Other					80 (25.2)

Intelligence

889 of these 1,477 patients had an adequate and tabulated assessment of their IQ. 69 of these 889 patients have an IQ greater than 110. A further 460 (51.7%) have a normal IQ (between 90 and 109). 89 (10%) are educable with an IQ between 80 and 89. Mild retardation (IQ 50–79) was present in 119 patients (13.4%). Severe retardation (IQ less than 50) occurred in 152 patients (17.1%). It was of interest that 14.8% of the Dandy-Walker syndrome patients and 9.5% of the patients with communicating hydrocephalus had an IQ greater than 110. Very few of the patients with aqueduct stenosis had an IQ greater than 110 and they accounted for the largest group of those with severe retardation.

Shunt Infection

287 of our 1,477 (19.4%) patients have had a shunt infection. However, these 1,477 patients have had 3,951 operative sessions indicating an infection rate per operative session of 7.3%. An operative session includes all operative maneuvers carried out at one time. This could include removal of one shunt and insertion of another shunt.

In the VP shunts, the infection rate per OR session was 7.7% compared to a 20.2% per patient infection rate. In the VA shunts the infection rate per OR session was 13.2% compared to a 35.4% per patient infection rate. In all fairness to the VA shunt we must point out that most of these shunts were inserted early on in this series when infection was a far commoner condition than it is in more recent years when most of the VP shunts were inserted.

The LP shunts fared best of all in terms of infection with a 2.8% infection rate per OR session and a 7.9% infection rate per patient. Of the infections, 29.2% occurred within 14 days of the surgical procedure on the shunt; a further 29.9% occurred between 14 and 28 days and only 12.2% occurred beyond 180 days. Although prophylactic antibiotics were used in a substantial number of patients in this series, because of the retrospective nature of the study we found it difficult to draw any definitive conclusions in regard to the efficacy of prophylactic antibiotics in reducing shunt infections. We are presently embarking on a double-blind study on a prospective basis to answer this question.

The commonest infecting organism was *Staphylococcus epidermidis* which accounted for 38.5% of the isolated organisms in shunts. *Staphylococcus aureus* came next and accounted for 17.9% of the organisms in infected shunts (table IV).

Conclusions

The modern treatment of hydrocephalus still remains far from ideal. Shunt obstruction and infection continue to be a source of significant morbidity and mortality. Better techniques and equipment have led to far better results. However, as this survey indicates there is still room for more improvement. The shunt-dependent child with aqueduct stenosis seems to fare worst of all with significant mortality as well as intellectual and neurological deficits. It is in this group of patients, where spontaneous arrest rarely occurs, that efforts to directly treat the CSF obstruction without the need of a by-pass shunt are imperative. At our institution in recent years we have been turning increasingly to percutaneous third ventriculostomy for this vulnerable group of patients with increasingly favorable results.

H.J. Hoffman, MD, Division of Neurosurgery, University of Toronto,
Hospital for Sick Children, Toronto (Canada)

Monogr. neural Sci., vol. 8, pp. 26–33 (Karger, Basel 1982)

Radiology of Shunt Complications in Childhood Hydrocephalus

Derek C. Harwood-Nash

Department of Radiology, The Hospital for Sick Children, Toronto, Ont., Canada

The assessment of shunt function and shunt complications by imaging techniques is provided by: (a) the physiological and 'anatomical' status of the shunt from the initial intracranial origin to the ultimate extracranial destination; (b) the patency of the shunt segments at the site of obstruction, and (c) early and late complications following its insertion. Furthermore, the cause of the obstruction can, in many cases, be determined as well as the effects of such an obstruction.

Within the Department of Medical Imaging at the Hospital for Sick Children, many modalities are available, each of which may be uniquely or concomitantly useful in the above assessment. A decision must be made as to what modality should be used and if multiple in what order, a diagnostic protocol. Such decisions must be controlled by the radiologist with direction by the neurosurgeon.

Investigative Protocol

The Shunt System Itself

Is It Obstructed and Where? The direct evidence is obtained by the use of radionuclide inserted into the system itself or within the CSF spaces and thence into the system. The site of a possible obstruction is then determined. Dislocation of the shunt position in part or in whole or a breach in continuity is provided by standard radiography.

Indirect evidence, other than the important clinical features provided by standard radiography and CT primarily (split sutures, enlarging ventricles, unusual shunt tip positions) and secondarily by nuclear medicine (e.g. encysted collections of CSF).

The Effects of Shunt Placement and Function

The position of the shunt tips are ascitated by standard radiography (of skull, chest and/or abdomen depending on shunt insertion sites). The *immediate* effects of the surgical intracranial insertion are best examined by CT (e.g. hemorrhage, immediate malposition). The *late* effects are examined according to that part of the body directed by clinical concern. Intracranial complications are best examined by CT (other than shunt position) e.g. for possible intracranial hemorrhage, ventricular enlargement, etc. Both intrathoracic and intra-abdominal complications, e.g. CSF encystments, are examined by standard radiography and possibly ultrasound in the abdomen for cystic masses. Extrusion of the shunts into the gastrointestinal tract may need barium studies or those in the cardiac pulmonary system, angiography.

Thus, the modalities that are primarily used are: function – nuclear medicine; shunt site – standard radiology; complications – CT (intracranial), standard radiology (extracranial). The particular clinical picture of each child will direct the initial and subsequent studies.

Radiological Features

These will be considered as applied to the investigation of shunt function, shunt position, and complications. The basic features of each are numerous and are listed in table I.

The commonest shunt performed at the Hospital for Sick Children is in the ventriculoperitoneal shunt, less commonly the lumboperitoneal shunt and rarely the ventriculo-atrial shunt. The frequency that these shunts malfunction (as a *first* shunt) is 34.7, 25, and 22.4%, respectively.

Shunt Malfunction

Shunt malfunction may be due to a block to the proximal and/or distal opening; failure of the reservoir valve system; discontinuity of the system as a whole; aberrant placement of the proximal or distal tips; tissue compartmentalization around the site of the proximal or distal tip.

The injection of a radionuclide ^{99m}-Tc DTPA into the valve itself (Gilday), using a 25-gauge needle, which with care and experience is not followed by destruction of the valve, enables reflux back into the ventricules, if patent, and drainage down the distal limb. The rapidity of drainage, possible sites of obstruction, or loculation around the peritoneal end are readily detected (fig. 1). The patency of the lumboperitoneal shunt is investigated by a lumbar puncture of the same radionuclide and imaging its passage in the peritoneum.

Discontinuity of the system as a whole is best determined (assuming the tubing is radiopaque) by standard PA radiographs of the chest and/or abdomen

Table I. Radiology of shunt complications

Shunt blockage	*Migration of shunt tip*	*Intra-abdominal complications*
Ventricular end	Cardiac end	peritonitis and adhesions
Ependymal impaction	transcaval	CSF peritoneal encystment
Choroid plexus plugging	transatrial	bowel obstruction
Intraventricular hemorrhage	intramyocardial position	bowel perforation
Inspissated brain tissue	transmyocardial position	*Intracranial complications*
Ventriculitis	pericardial effusion	intracranial hemorrhage from insertion
Disconnection	disconnection into pulmonary artery	ventriculitis
Cardiac end	peritoneal end	subdural hematoma
Thrombosis	gastric perforation	extradural hematoma
Superior vena cava malposition	intestinal perforation	CSF hygroma
Right ventricular malposition	transrectal emergence	upward brain stem herniation
Disconnection	transumbilical emergence	*Intraspinal complications*
Bacterial colonization	intrahernial coiling	arachnoiditis
Intraluminal shunt debris	*Infection and thrombosis*	scoliosis
Valcular dysfunction	cardiac end	cauda equina abnormalities
Peritoneal end	septicemia	neurological abnormalities
Omental plugging	pneumonia	*Miscellaneous*
Peritoneal adhesion	pulmonary infarcts and abscesses	congestive cardiac failure
Lumbar end	cor pulmonale	shunt glomerulonephritis
Nerve root plugging	tricuspid vegetations and incompetence	inappropriate ADH secretion
Adhesions	superior vena cava thrombosis	extracranial malignant metastases
Pleural end		shunt dependency
Adhesions		foramen magnum syndrome
Impactions		
Extrapleural or lung		

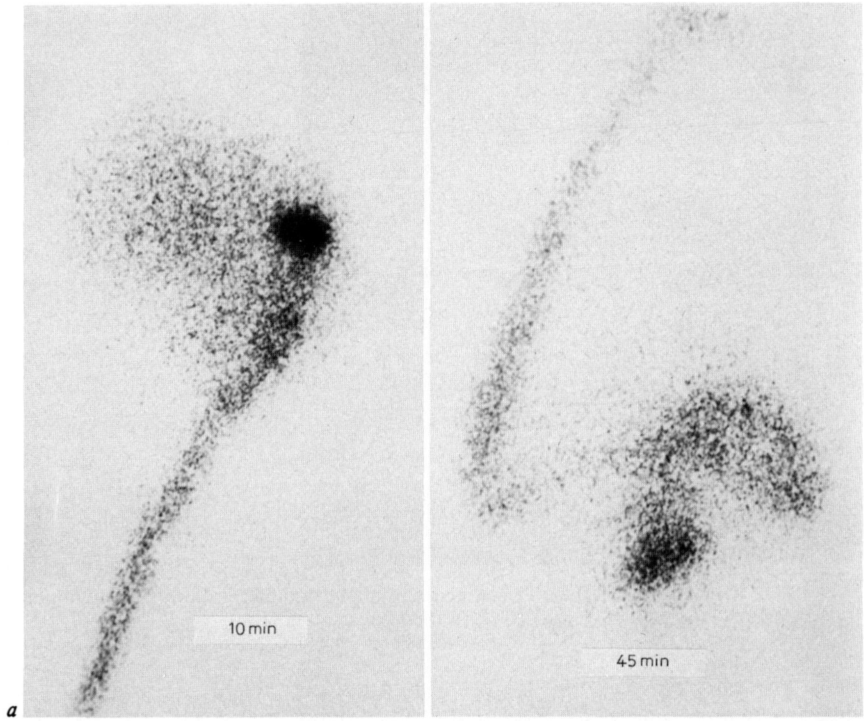

Fig. 1. Peritoneal block. (*a*) At 10 min there is reflux into the ventricles from the reservoir and at 45 min (*b*) the distal peritoneal end shows blockage with encystment of the radionuclide in the peritoneal cavity.

and a lateral skull radiograph. Such discontinuity is commonest at the junction of the ventricular catheter and the reservoir.

Shunt Position

Aberrant placement of the proximal tip is usually within the temporal horn, third ventricle via the foramen of Monro, within the brain tissue or the midline interhemispheric fissure. All result in poorly functioning shunts. It is common to see the shunt cross the midline yet function well. The distal tip may be primarily misplaced within the abdominal wall, elsewhere in the thoracic cardiovascular system than the middle of the right atrium, within lung tissue if a pleural shunt, etc. Secondarily, the shunt may retract away from the previously optimal site by patient growth. All these positions are detectable by standard radiography. A posterior-anterior and lateral skull radiograph is performed with a localization of

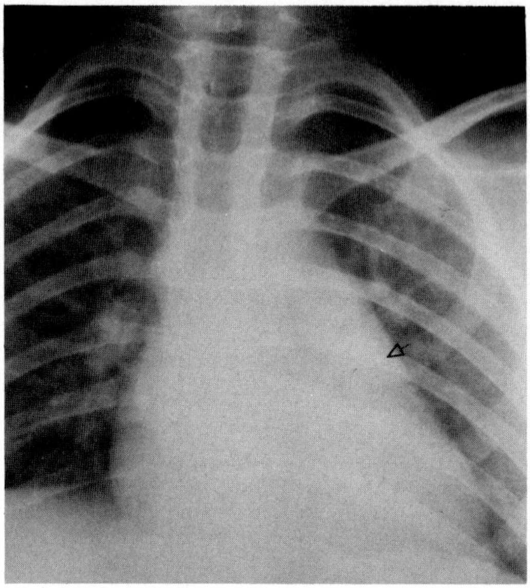

Fig. 2. Detached cathether. The cardiac end of the catheter is detached and has migrated into a left pulmonary vein (arrow).

the proximal cranial end. Wire-strengthened catheters may erode through virtually anything, bowel wall, umbilicus, scrotum, etc.

Peritoneal encystment around the distal tip may occur and may be seen by ultrasound or radiography as a large intra-abdominal mass. Furthermore, the CSF may be poorly absorbed by the mesentry and bowel and result in a CSF peritoneal effusion. The obstruction may be relative due to an increased production of CSF as seen in the rare choroid plexus papilloma. Similar location may occur at the pleural distal end.

Detachment of the distal end, if in the right atrium may pass up the main pulmonary artery and out into a pulmonary branch. Its retrieval may be accomplished, after a pulmonary angiography, by percutaneous femoral vein catheterization. A guide wire with a distal basket is passed up the catheter and snares the shunt catheter and withdraws it back through the femoral vein and a sleeve (fig. 2).

The presence of a shunt in good position and mildly or moderately enlarged ventricles does not necessarily mean the shunt is blocked. Inadvertent too rapid a collapse of the ventricles is danger. It is the progressive increase in ventricular size that objectively identifies a blocked shunt. Contrariwise, however, small ventricles do denote a functioning shunt with the exception of the slit-like ventricles with thickened ependymal walls that are relatively rigid. These will be discussed later. It has been stated, however, that 87% of patients with enlarging or enlarged ventricles had improperly functioning shunts as determined clinically and by improper pumping. 93% of patients with normal or small ventricles had a functioning shunt.

Complications

Complications result *immediately* from the insertion of the shunt other than simply malposition or mainly intracranial and from the positioning of the proximal shunt catheter. Perforation of an intra-abdominal viscus is extremely rare. These are investigated by CT and the majority are inadvertent intracranial hemorrhage usually intracerebral. These are usually minimal and rarely result in significant clinical signs or sequelae. Immediate subdural hematomas are rare.

Late complications are more common. The most common used to be subdural hematomas due to rapid shrinkage of the ventricles and tearing of the bridging veins due to a concomitant shrinkage of the brain as a whole away from the inner table. This occurred due to low-pressure valve reservoirs or direct drainage. High-pressure valves have obviated these to a certain extent (fig. 3). Infections present as ventriculitis in particular, meningitis or rarely abscesses. CT is the procedure of choice for all these complications. Meningitis per se is difficult to detect on CT. Loculations of one or more of the ventricles (fig. 4), and/or the development of porencephalic cysts is more common, in particular the lateral ventricle or fourth ventricle. These usually occur after multiple and often infected shunts. Ventricular bands are often seen on CT or multiple porencephalic cysts.

The possible patency of the ventricular pathways and/or cysts is best examined in conjunction with CT by the insertion of 1 ml of isotonic metrizamide into the ventricle or cavity directly or via a shunt. This small concentration is easily detected on the CT scan. This is a significant and useful aid in planning of future shunts and revisions. The passage of this metrizamide or the lack of same is easily detected from cavity to cavity.

Irregular small slit-like ventricles often with thickened ependymal wall represent the 'slit ventricle syndrome or shunt dependency state' (fig. 5) whereby clinical deterioration may occur rapidly in children often with thickened skulls and closed not fused sutures. These ventricles can be likened to cavities with rigid walls with no compliancy. Irregular occipital horns and slit frontal horns are frequent CT findings. Subtemporal decompression is advocated as shunt replacement is difficult. Scoliosis in children, after lumboperitoneal shunts, was a problem previously when silastic tubes shunts were used. However, better shunt material now obviates this but severe scoliosis and very irregular lumbar subarachnoid spaces on myelography was seen.

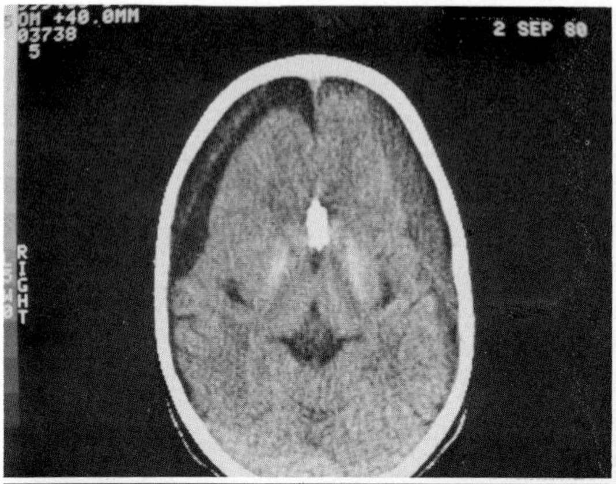

3

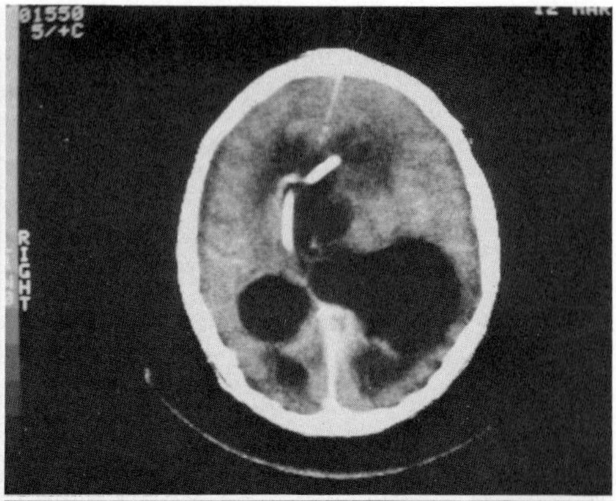

4a

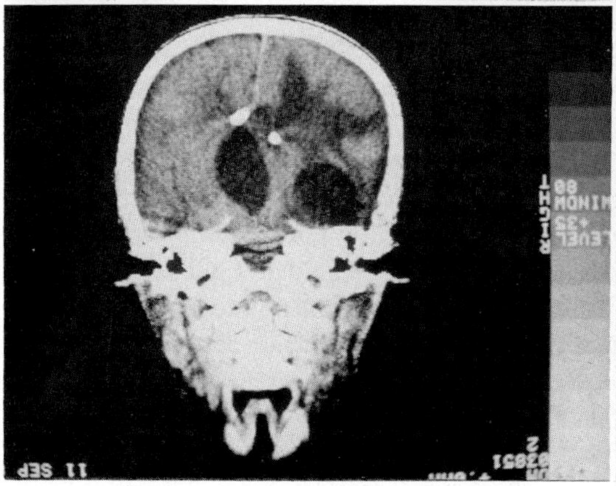

4b

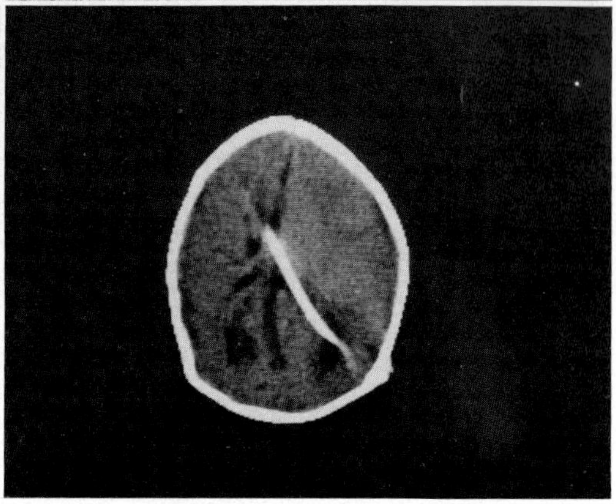

5

Fig. 3. Subdural hematomas. Bilateral frontoparietal subdural hematomas of differing ages due to rapid decompression of enlarged ventricles by shunting.

Fig. 4. Ventricular loculations. An axial (*a*) and a coronal (*b*) view shows multiple shunts with encystment of the left lateral ventricle posteriorly and of the third ventricle due to ventriculitis.

Fig. 5. Slit-like ventricles. Shunting resulting in slit-like ventricles with slightly dilated occipital horns.

Conclusion

Any child in whom a shunt dysfunction or complication is suspected clinically, or by attempted manual pumping or the reservoir, should have standard radiography (PA and lateral views of the skull, anteroposterior view of the abdomen and/or chest depending on the site of the distal end). If the distal end is in the chest a lateral radiograph should also be performed, using a very fast exposure time to capture the image of the tip within the fast beating heart. Nuclear medicine is a procedure of choice for the assessment of function and blockage. CT should be used for any suspect intracerebral abnormality or for ventricular size and combined with metrizamide if loculation of the ventricles and/or formation of porencephalic cysts is suspected.

D.C. Harwood-Nash, MD, Department of Radiology, The Hospital for Sick Children, Toronto, Ont. (Canada)

Monogr. neural Sci., vol. 8, pp. 34–38 (Karger, Basel 1982)

Quantitative Measurement of Cerebrospinal Fluid Shunt Flow

Osamu Sato[a], *Masaki Ohya*[a], *Ryuichi Tsugane*[a], *Katsumi Ikei*[b], *Yutaka Suzuki*[b]

[a]Departments of Neurosurgery and [b]Radiology, Tokai University, School of Medicine Bohsei-Dai, Isehara, Japan

Introduction

Treatments of hydrocephalus with a valve-regulated shunt has the highest complication rate in neurosurgical practice. One of the problems we have in shunt surgery is an obstruction of the system, and this could cause a critical status in many instances. Under the usual circumstances, a diagnosis of shunt patency is made by checking the response of the flushing device to digital compression or patient's clinical picture. However, at the same time, the finding of this digital palpation of the reservoir and its neurological status has never been appreciated as a truly reliable sign to indicate whether the shunting system is properly functioning or not [6]. Furthermore, in contrast to the shunt obstruction, cerebrospinal fluid overdrainage phenomena through the system could cause low-pressure headaches, upward displacement of the brain stem and slit-like ventricles which might induce intolerance to minimal pressure rises leading to a real disaster [2]. In avoidance of these misleading informations and undesirable outcomes, the treatment of hydrocephalus with a shunting device would get close to its final goal.

The purpose of this paper is to describe a simple technique for injecting a small amount of a radioactive substance into the shunt reservoir to assess patency and the rate of cerebrospinal fluid flow of the shunt system through which the extracranial diversion of cerebrospinal fluid is made for hydrocephalus of various pathogeneses.

Method

A multicrystal gamma camera (Baird Atomic System 70) was the device used to measure the radionuclide activity. The whole system consists of collimeters, magnetic disk,

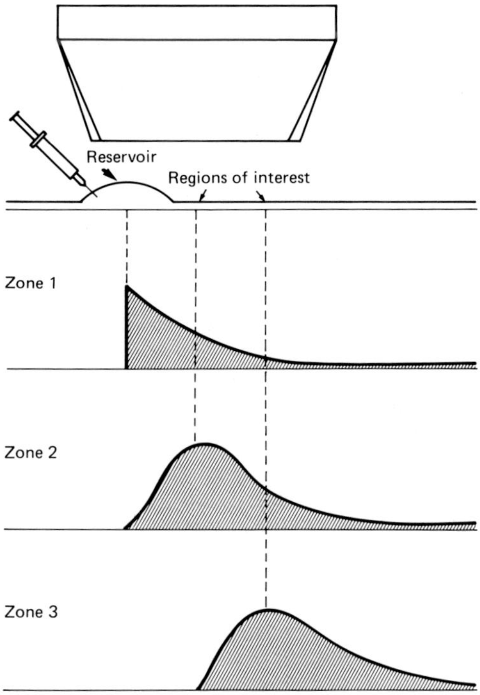

Fig. 1. The schematic illustration of the principle used for the measurement of cerebrospinal fluid shunt flow.

computer, cathode ray tube and operating table. A total number of 294 crystal collimeters provided a wide range coverage as a detector. Prior to its clinical application, preliminary experiments were done to estimate some possible errors in the measurement of flow rates using this method. With the ventricular catheter being connected to an infusion pump, 200–500 μCi of technetium pertechnetate in a volume of 0.02–0.03 ml was introduced into the flushing device as a bolus. The small volume was chosen so that volume displacement per se would alter the shunt dynamics as little as possible. Saline infusion rates varied from 0.012 to 0.617 ml/min and immediate images of radioactivity along the entire tubing system were obtained with the gamma camera which was connected to a magnetic disk and a computer. The recording was made at 1- or 3-s intervals and continued for 5 min for fast flow rates and 20 min for slow flow rates. From the area over the flushing device and two regions of interest along the distal tubing, the time/activity curves were visualized on a display cathode ray tube and printed out on recording paper through the computer. Zone 1 shows the time/activity curve from the flushing device, and its activity decreases gradually as time passes and zones 2 and 3 indicate the time/activity curves from the two points along the distal tubing and the time difference between two peaks is the expression of the movement of the fluid in the catheter (fig. 1). Deducting 30% from each peak count of two

Table I.

Case No.	Age, years	Etiology	Shunt system	Valve palpation	Flow rate, ml/min	Ventricular size	Symptom	Follow-up
1	1	congenital	V-A.PM	normal	0.03	moderate		
2	1 month	meningocele	V-P, PH	normal	very slow	moderate	+	
3	1	meningocele	V-P, PH	obstruct.	0	moderate		arrested
4	3	4th vent. tumor	V-P, DC	slow-fill	0.15[a]	slit-like		revised
5	10	4th vent. tumor	V-P, DC	normal	0.16	slit-like		
6	2	frontal tumor	V-P, PL	normal	0.29	moderate		
7	6	frontal tumor	V-P, PM	normal	0.21	moderate		
8	3	post-meningitis	V-P, PM	normal	0.09	marked	+	revised
		post-meningitis	+ slits	normal	0.60	moderate		
9	62	ventricular	V-P, PL	normal	0.06	normal		
		hemorrhage	V-P, PL	slow-fill.	0.09	slit-like	+	+ASV
			V-P + ASV	normal	very slow	normal		
10	69	post-trauma	V-P, DC	normal	0.33	moderate		
11	60	post-SAH	V-P, DC	normal	0.25	moderate		
12	37	post-SAH	V-P, PM	normal	0.07[a]	moderate		arrested
13	58	post-SAH	V-P, DC	normal	0.10	normal		
14	46	post-SAH	V-P, PM	normal	0.13	normal		
15	48	post-SAH	V-P, DC	obstruct.	0	moderate		revised
			V-P, DC	normal	0.33	normal		
16	72	post-SAH	L-P, DC	normal	0.02	marked	+	revised
		post-SAH	V-P, DC	normal	0.10	marked		
17	65	C-p angle tumor	V-P, PM	normal	0.05	moderate		

P = Pudenz; H = high pressure; M = medium pressure; L = low pressure; DC = Dow Corning (Ames design).
[a] Irregular flow pattern.

regions of interest, mean transit times are calculated. The difference between these two values is called a 'peak-to-peak time', T. A simple formula: $F = \pi R^2 L/T$ provides flow rate, where R is the radius of the tube and L is the known distance of two regions of interest. In conclusion of this experimental work, the possible error of the flow rates calculated was estimated as 10% when the actual flow rates were set between 0.1 and 0.6 ml/min; however, it increased up to 30 or 40% when the actual flow rates were less than 0.033 ml/min.

Clinical Application

It is easily understood that cerebrospinal fluid flow rate through the shunt varies greatly as the patient's posture changes; therefore, the patient was kept in a supine position more than 60 min prior to the examination. A summary of clinically applied cases is shown in table I. Recent data from a CT scan, findings on shunt valve digital palpation, and the clinical picture were also recorded. The patient's head was kept flat and the collimeters were set parallel to the plane of the catheter as much as possible.

Case Report A

A 10-year-old boy who was operated on the fourth ventricle tumor and the ventricular system reduced its size following VP shunt. The shunting system appeared to be working properly and the time/activity curves were expressed as smooth figures and the peaks did shift from zone 2 to zone 3. The flow rate was calculated as 0.16 ml/min.

Case Report B

This is a case of non-communicating hydrocephalus which developed following intraventricular hemorrhage. A VP shunt was installed with a Pudenz low-pressure valve; however, the patient's condition deteriorated gradually and finally became apathetic. On palpation of the valve, malfunction of the system was suggested without good refill of the flushing device after being compressed. There was a flow rate of 0.09 ml/min in spite of no good recovery of the flushing device and the CT scan demonstrated so-called slit-like ventricles.

Case Report C

This is a case of medulloblastoma. A radioisotope which was injected into the reservoir demonstrated a temporary stasis and the activity decreased extremely slowly. This intermittent flow had the rate of 0.15 ml/min and this sort of irregular flow pattern was also observed in another case. Both of these developed shunt obstruction within 1–3 months following the tests. The flow rate itself appeared within its normal limit but this kind of reluctance of flow would be the indication of the impending shunt obstruction.

Case Report D

This is a 1-month-old boy who had an occipital meningocele and the aqueductal stenosis. A VP shunt was put in place with a Pudenz high-pressure valve; however, he continued to have a tense fontanel and the head size remained the same. A large amount of the radioactivity stayed in the flushing device even 10 min after its introduction while a pumping maneuver of the flushing device revealed a good cerebrospinal fluid flow through the distal catheter. It was concluded that the high-pressure valve was inadequate in this case and the valve was replaced with a low-pressure valve when his condition improved with now a well-functioning shunting system.

Discussion

Reviewing these results, the important thing is the judgement of cases in which clinical improvement is not quite as satisfactory as expected after shunt tubing being installed. In most cases with shunt malfunction, shunt flow rates were shown to be less than 0.1 ml/min and from our experience, though still limited, it could be stated that the shunt function would be quite adequate when the flow rates are between 0.1 and 0.3 ml/min with a smooth decreasing pattern of the radioisotope activity in the reservoir. As a classical method in determining whether or not a shunt system is patent, valvography has been frequently used and this method would tell us the site of the obstruction as well, if there is any [1]. Also the detection of cerebrospinal fluid flow in the shunt tube by cold transfer has been documented as a decent method for its harmless way [3]. However, these are not quantitative in measuring the flow and it has been recognized nowadays as rather a critical matter not only to discern patency of the shunt installed but also to recognize its actual flow rate through the system. Not being a measure of the clearance curve of the radioactivity injected into the reservoir [4, 5], the problem of incomplete mixing of the material due to a complex streamline in the reservoir is avoided; therefore, this is a particularly attractive technique in its simple way accounting for a direct cerebrospinal fluid flow rate through the shunting system.

References

1 Amador, L.V.; Jara, O.; Porras, C.L.: Valvography: a test for patency of Holter valve shunts. Am. J. Dis. Child. *117:* 190–193 (1969).

2 Faulhauer, K.; Schmitz, P.: Overdrainage phenomena in shunt treated hydrocephalus. Acta neurochir. *45:* 89–101 (1978).

3 Go, G.; Van Der Veen, P.H.; Van Den Berg, J.W.: Detection of CSF flow in ventriculo-atrial shunts by cold transfer, Devl. Med. Child Neur. *12:* suppl., pp. 69–72 (1970).

4 Harbert J.; Haddad D.; McCullough, D.: Quantitation of cerebrospinal fluid shunt flow. Nucl. Med. *112:* 379–387 (1974).

5 Maeda, T.; Mori, H.; Hisada, K.; Kadoya, S.: Evaluation of cerebrospinal fluid flow through a Pudenz 12 mm or a standard Rickham reservoir: phantom experiments. Investve Radiol. *12:* 555–558 (1977).

6 Osaka, K.; Yamasaki, S.; Hirayama, A.; Sato, N.; Ohi, Y.; Matsumoto, S.: Correlation of the response of the flushing device to compression with the clinical picture in the evaluation of the functional status of the shunting system. Child's Brain *3:* 25–30 (1977).

O. Sato, MD, Departments of Neurosurgery, Tokai University, School of Medicine, Bohsei-Dai, Isehara, Kanagawa 259–11 (Japan)

Monogr. neural Sci., vol. 8, pp. 39–42 (Karger, Basel 1982)

Radionuclide Imaging Shuntography for the Evaluation of Shunt Patency

Barry N. French, Marilyn Swanson
University of California, Davis Medical Center, Sacramento, Calif., USA

Patency of a cerebrospinal fluid shunt system can be demonstrated by making serial images on a scintillation camera of the migration of radioactive tracer injected into the shunt reservoir. The majority of reports suggest that passage of isotope from injection site to distal drainage site is equivalent to adequate function of the shunt. However, patency is not always synonymous with adequate function of the shunt system.

Material

The study consisted of a retrospective review of a personal series of 43 shunted, hydrocephalic children undergoing 78 radionuclide imaging shuntograms (RNIS) performed to evaluate the patency of their cerebrospinal fluid (CSF) shunts. The patients are relatively selected in that children with obvious shunt obstruction determined by clinical features, CT scan and plain roentgenograms did not have RNIS performed. The etiology of the hydrocephalus was associated with spinal dysraphism in 20 patients and attributed to meningitis in 6, to a congenital cyst in 5, to intraventricular hemorrhage of prematurity in 4, to trauma in 1, and to idiopathic causes in 7 patients. The anatomical type of hydrocephalus was communicating in 5 patients, obstructive in 10, related to the Arnold-Chiari malformation in 20, and was unknown in 8 patients. These 43 patients underwent 78 shuntograms. 70 shuntograms were performed on ventriculoperitoneal shunt systems, and 8 on ventriculoatrial systems. 12 shuntograms were done in patients with double cranial reservoirs connected to a single peritoneal catheter by a 'Y' connector. The types of reservoir punctured for the shuntograms were Pudenz in 67 instances, Holter in 3, Rickham in 4, Mischler in 2 and in 1 instance each, an Ames and a multipurpose system.

Method

The isotope used for 74 of the shuntograms was ^{99m}-Tc pertechnetate in a dose ranging from 0.5 to 3 mCi in a volume usually less than 1 ml. Four studies utilized ^{111}-In diethylenetriaminepentaacetate (DPTA) in similar doses and volumes. A Nuclear-Chicago Pho/Gamma HP scintillation camera equipped with a low-energy, high-sensitivity colimator, was used to obtain sequential 100,000 count images over the course of the shunt system. The camera was calibrated for the 140-keV photopeak of ^{99m}-Tc using a 20% window. In the four instances in which ^{111}-In DPTA was used, the camera was calibrated for the 190-keV photopeak. All patients are placed in the supine position initially. The scalp over the reservoir is clean-shaven, prepared with Betadine and draped. The scalp is nicked with a large needle which is then discarded. A number 23 needle on a syringe penetrates into the reservoir through the nicked area to prevent taking a core of epithelium within the hollow needle. The peritoneal portion of the chamber is entered unless specific information regarding the ventricles is desired. The ventricular pressure is measured with a standard manometer from a lumbar puncture tray and 2 or 3 ml of CSF is removed for culture, glucose, protein, and cell count and differential. All shuntograms were performed by reservoir puncture with the exception of two studies performed by ventricular puncture. The isotope is then injected gently into the reservoir and the distribution of the radioactivity is observed on the persistence scope of the scintillation counter to ensure the activity enters the reservoir and the shunt tubing rather than extravasating. The abdomen is scanned immediately to rule out direct injection of the isotope throughout the length of the catheter. Subsequently, sequential pictures of 100,000 counts each are taken over the cranium, neck, thorax and abdominal cavity to record spontaneous passage of isotope distally into the peritoneal cavity (early supine patency). If spontaneous migration is not demonstrated after 10 min in the supine position (delayed supine patency), the patient is held erect and immediately rescanned to detect spontaneous migration of the isotope distally (immediate erect patency). If no migration occurs over 10 min, the reservoir is pumped to assess mechanical passage of the isotope (pump patency). In the event that the diffusion of the isotope in the abdomen is not rapidly widespread, delayed images are taken to demonstrate possible distal catheter encystment. Patients with double cranial reservoirs require a separate injection of isotope into each reservoir to confirm patency of both limbs of the system.

Results and Discussion

The shuntogram was considered accurate if no symptoms developed and if no revision was required for 6 months after the test indicated a patent shunt; or if an obstruction was confirmed at an operation after the shuntogram indicated a malfunctioning shunt. A shuntogram was considered inaccurate if a shunt revision was required to relieve persistent symptoms within 6 months of a test indicating patency of the shunt system. In such situations, the shuntogram was deemed to have shown deceptive patency. The flow patterns that indicated patency of the shunt system and that best correlated with adequate shunt function were early or delayed supine patency (fig. 1) and immediate erect patency. These patterns demonstrate spontaneous flow, as opposed to flow generated by pumping the reservoir. Pump patency did not correlate with adequate shunt function (table I). In 48 studies that proved spontaneous patency of the shunt, there were 14 studies (29%) in which the shuntogram was considered to be deceptive because the clinical problem was not explained. In each case, the clinical features and other investigations led to the diagnosis of shunt malfunction. 19 shuntograms

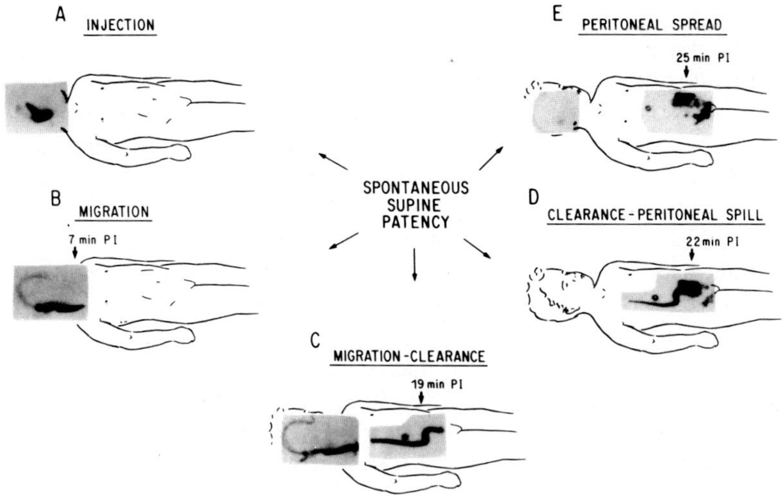

Fig. 1. Radionuclide imaging shuntography demonstrating spontaneous supine patency.

Table I.

Isotope pattern	Number of studies (76)[1]	Adequate patency	Deceptive patency	Obstruction
Early supine patency	11	8	3	–
Delayed supine patency	25	15	10	–
Immediate erect patency	12	11	1	–
Delayed erect patency	4	0	4	–
Pump patency	5	0	5	–
Obstruction	19	0	0	19

[1] Extravasation occurred in 2 studies that are not included in the table.

were interpreted as complete obstruction of the shunt system. The test accurately indicated obstruction in all 19 cases with no instances of deceptive information.

The more frequent situations in which deceptive patency occurs are the intermittently functioning shunt, the incompletely obstructed shunt, and the provision of incomplete anatomical information about the CSF pathways. Intermittent functioning of a shunt frequently occurs in the setting of exceedingly small ventricles in which periodic coaptation of the ventricular walls obstructs the ventricular catheter but function may be normal at other times. Incomplete obstruction of the shunt system may occur at the proximal or distal ends or somewhere in between. The process is usually associated with an elevated opening pressure of the shunt system such that the patient's intraventricular pressure rises to symptomatic levels. However, CSF drainage through the system still occurs and the shuntogram will indicate patency. In some patients, a shunt system may be functioning well but symptoms are produced by another intracranial lesion such as a subdural hematoma, undiagnosed tumor or cyst or entrapment of a portion of the ventricular system. The shuntogram will indicate adequate function of the shunt but may not clarify the intracranial pathology. Three studies in our series fell into this group. 1 patient had entrapment of the lateral ventricle, another had encystment of the fourth ventricle, and the third patient had a noncommunicating basal arachnoid cyst.

B.N. French, MD, University of California, Davis Medical Center, Sacramento, CA (USA)

Monogr. neural Sci., vol. 8, pp. 43–47 (Karger, Basel 1982)

Bihemispheric Transcephalic Impedanciometry during Infancy

Abraham Krivoy, Jaime Krivoy, Mauricio Krivoy

Servicio de Neurocirugía, Hospital de Niños J.M. de Los Ríos, Caracas, Venezuela

Introduction

After the communication of *Reigel et al.* [8], we became interested in the method of transcephalic impedanciometry because, together with the cephalic diaphanoscopy, within the first year of life, both are easy methods in screening patients and, in particular, the transcephalic impedance is sensitive to evaluate the shunt treatment and its failure.

Van Harreveld et al. [10] demonstrated that the value of cerebral impedance changed in accordance to the watery contents of the brain. *Jarzembsky* [2] demonstrated the modifications of electrical current in the brain during application of diffuse electrical currents. *Robinson and Tomkins* [9] used the impedance method for localizing brain structures.

Method

We found that the Siemen's Direkt Reograph 933, which was not built for this purpose, is useful for the transcephalic impedance measurement. The output impedance of the amplifier is 2 × 100 kΩ using a cascade circuit. Measure of current source: square-wave approximately 30 kHz with 20 V and 1 mA each channel. The reading of the resistance is made in two analogue milli-amperimeters calibrated in ohms from 0 to 100 Ω. The Reograph is powered by 110 V 60 cycles AC current of line connection. We used 6 silver Nihon Kohden Ne 113 S electrodes, 1 cm diameter and 3 mm thickness. The two central electrodes for current application are placed 2 cm above nasion and inion. The other four electrodes for voltage measurement are placed 2.5 cm laterally to the two central electrodes (fig. 1).

The skin where the electrodes are placed should be scrubbed with a mild abrasive soap and dried. The electrodes are filled with bentonite, the usual electrolytic paste in EEG, which keeps the electrodes in place or you can use the EKG paste with a supporting rubber strip around the head.

The contact resistance requires to be between 4,000 and 10,000 Ω in order to

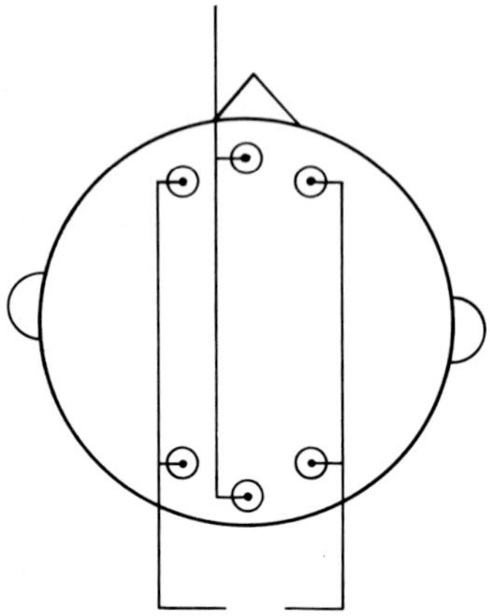

Fig. 1. Graphic representing the central pair of electrodes for current application located 2.5 cm above the nasion and inion. Two lateral pairs of electrodes for measurement of voltage are placed 2.5 cm laterally to the current electrodes.

reproduce the measurment of the impedance. Due to the fact that when using the Reograph it is easy to manually swith the voltage electrode leads from one side to the other, it is then possible to verify the reproducibility of the values in both hemispheres.

The impedance measurements were performed in 140 cases under 36 months of age, 7 cases of convulsive disorders, 7 of macrocephaly, 5 with scaphocephaly, and 1 with mental retardation, all of their values were normal. 2 other cases were meningitis, 2 had posterior fossa tumors, 9 with trauma, 5 with myelomeningocele, 1 with hydranencephaly, 1 with microcephaly, 31 hydrocephalus, and 4 with an obstructed shunt, 1 porencephaly and 3 cerebral atrophy. 65 cases were normal.

Results

Normal Infants. 65 normal infants were evaluated in our series, 37 of whom were selected because they proceeded from normal pregnancy and delivery and had a normal weight at birth; 29 of them were followed until 7 months of age and only 8 up to the first year. At birth we found a transcephalic symmetric impedance ranging from 28 to 40 Ω, with an average of 34 Ω and a standard deviation of 4.76, and a monthly increase of 4 Ω. At 12 months the values reached an average of 86.67 Ω with a standard deviation of 11.55 Ω. From 12 months on, the reliability of the methods decrease, but it could be still a good one if the value found is inferior to 80 Ω in both or one hemisphere corroborated by switching the voltage cables of the electrodes.

Macrocephaly. 7 cases referred for evaluation with percentiles greater than 98% showed a normal impedance; computerized axial tomography (CAT) was also normal.

Meningitis. From 2 cases of meningitis, at 5 and 14 months old, respectively, the latter showed a low impedance value (66 Ω) which was followed during treatment by an improvement of the clinical features and impedance values within a period of 10 days. We can only speculate about an exudative phase, or transient hydrocephaly during meningitis as the cause of the low impedance.

Posterior Fossa Tumor. In 2 cases, 1 of them 2 years old with 74 Ω and the other 3 years old with 60 Ω, both had low values due to their secondary ventricular enlargement verified by CAT scan.

Trauma. 3 of 9 cases showed low values with an improvement parallel to their clinical features which became normal within the following 6 weeks.

Myolomeningocele. 4 of 5 cases studied showed low values, with normal cephalic circumference but with ventricular enlargement verified by CAT scan.

Hydranencephaly. 1 case 5 months old with 12 Ω.

Hydrocephaly. 31 cases showed low impedance values, with an improvement within a few weeks after the shunting; 4 of them with valvular dysfunction relapsed to low values and following the revision they again reached normal values.

Porencephaly. 1 case with abnormal asymmetric values.

Unilateral Cerebral Atrophy. 3 cases with asymmetry in their abnormal impedance value.

Discussion

Inasmuch as the measurement of the variations of the transcephalic impedance (ΔZ) due to the variation of blood pulsation passing through the brain, called reoencephalography [3–7], is a more sophisticated and delicate method than the simple measurement of all the impedance of the brain, we have used the same device built for reoencephalography because, as *Reigel et al.* [8] pointed out, we coupled the electrodes with a high-impedance constant current source and two voltmeters connected in parallel, keeping a fixed distance between the electrodes. We use 30-kHz square wave current, the same used in reoencephalography.

The term bihemispheric used in the title depends on the constant asymmetrical values we have found in some cases with asymmetrical collection of fluid, like porencephaly, unilateral subdural collection, and asymmetrical cerebral atrophy, verified by CAT, ventriculography, or any other method, either combined or alone. For that reason, in some experiments about the electrical transmission in the brain, we suggest that it follows an onion-shaped pattern like figure 2, and that is the reason why we can speak about lateralization of the

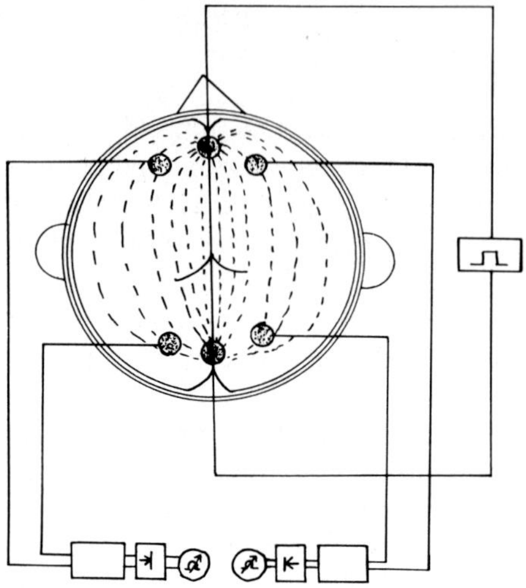

Fig. 2. Onion pattern of current distribution between the two central electrodes, according to which asymmetrical values in asymmetrical pathology is possible as the Driscoll [1] spherical model has indicated.

lesion or fluid accumulation when values are constantly asymmetric. Probably this explanation is very similar to the one described by *Driscoll* [1] in the spherical model of the distribution of the current applied to the head, which states that when there are internal alterations in resistance, a redistribution of the current flow will occur.

References

1 Driscoll, D.A.; Theoretical model of the human head with applications of current flow calculations and EEG interpretaion; thesis, Burlington (1970).
2 Jarzembski, W.; Electrical current in the brain during application of diffuse electrical currents; thesis, Milwaukee (1971).
3 Krivoy, A.: Reoencefalografía. Centro Médico *46:* 87–97 (1974).
4 Krivoy, A.: Aspectos biofísicos de la reoencefalografía y del comportamiento del tejido sanguíneo. Centro Medico *53:* 15–25 (1976).
5 Krivoy, A.: Consideraciones clínicas del valor de la onda derivada en la reoencefalografía. Presentado en la Academia Nacional de Medicina, 1974.
6 Krivoy, A.: Lo nuevo en el diagnóstico neurológico: la reoencefalografía por impedancia. Trib. med. Venezuela *2:* 29–32 (1976).
7 Nyboyer, J.: Electrical impedance plethysmography; 2nd ed. (Thomas, Springfield (1970).

8 Reigel, D.H.; Dallma, D.E.; Scarff, T.B.; Woodford, J.: Transcephalic impedance measurement during infancy. Devl. Med. Child Neur. *19:* 295–304 (1977).
9 Robinson, B.W.; Tomkins, H.E.: Impedance method for localizing brain structures. Arch. Neurol., Chicago *10:* 563–574 (1964).
10 Van Harreveld, A., Hooper, N.K., Cusick, J.T. Brain electrolytes and cortical impedance. Am. J. Physiol. *187:* 180–192 (1961).

Dr. Abraham Krivoy O, Avda. Manuel Felipe Tovar, Qta. Hopsing 54–1,
San Bernardino 1101, Caracas (Venezuela)

Monogr. neural Sci., vol. 8, p. 48 (Karger, Basel 1982)

Value of CT in the Shunted Pediatric Patient

M. Judith Donovan Post[a], *Larry K. Page*[b],

[a]Division of Neuroradiology, Department of Radiology and [b]Department of Neurological Surgery at the University of Miami School of Medicine, Miami, Fla., USA

Because of the advent of CT, the shunted pediatric patient can now be evaluated at routine invervals in a safe, comfortable, and relatively non-invasive manner. Due to the ability of CT to discriminate CSF from surrounding brain parenchyma and therefore to assess ventricular size, ventriculography and angiography can often be avoided in the child suspected of having a malfunctioning shunt.

A review of the CT scans performed recently at the University of Miami School of Medicine on the shunted pediatric patient with symptoms and signs of raised intracranial pressure has verified the reliability of CT in assessing shunt malfunction and has shown that the need for more invasive studies is obviated in the majority of patients.

Our study indicated that CT was valuable in assessing the shunted pediatric patient because it could: (1) assess the position of the shunt tube; (2) determine ventricular size; (3) discern causes of shunt malfunction unrelated to an extraventricular position of the shunt tube (such as septation and multiloculation of the ventricles); (4) demonstrate shunt-related complications (such as subdural, intraparenchymal and/or intraventricular hematomas, ventriculitis, and encephalomalacic cavities or tracts), and (5) uncover etiologies of raised intracranial pressure other than shunt malfunction (as expanding subarachnoid cysts, enlarging tumors, and inflammatory lesions).

Clues for the presence of shunt malfunction provided by CT scans in the study included: (1) improper position of the shunt tube; (2) large ventricles; (3) an increase in ventricular size over prior studies; (4) a change in ventricular configuration; (5) transexudation of CSF from the frontal horns, and (6) accumulation of CSF in the subcutaneous soft tissues about the shunting device. Only in a small proportion of patients, such as those with ventricular fibrosis and those with thin cortical mantles, was the CT scan not diagnostic of shunt malfunction or of shunt patency.

M.J.D. Post, MD, Division of Neuroradiology, Department of Radiology, University of Miami School of Medicine, Miami, FL (USA)

Monogr. neural Sci., vol. 8, pp. 49–51 (Karger, Basel 1982)

Mechanical Problems in Shunts

Ervin Paraicz
National Institute of Neurosurgery, Budapest, Hungary

My task would be to enumerate and summarize the mechanical complications of the different shunt systems; this list is rather long.

Let us first see the older parts of the list (fig. 1) – the complications of ventriculoatrial shunts. Do you still remember the more than 50 old methods that have failed to yield lasting results? This was at the time when the first encouraging reports about venous shunts just reached us. But, soon enough, we became aware of the great number of complications. Then we decided to approach the problem from a different angle, namely how to treat the presenting complications. Numerous participants of this section had elaborated new methods to improve the outcome (treatment of septic complications, preventive antibiotic measures with respect to shunts and the operative field, the control of free flow with isotope, ICP monitoring, the techniques for surgical revision, etc.). Another direction, prophylactic measures, has been elaborated to prevent complications. Because in the heart the obstruction of the distal catheter was but rarely encountered, and most of the time the catheter retracted in the veins became occluded, some investigators recommended the prophylactic lengthening of the cardiac catheter before a passage disturbance in the shunt could develop. A telescopic shunt was constructed in the hope that it would be suitable to keep pace with the growing body of the patients. The children with shunt operation were put on regular heparin therapy in order to avoid thrombosis development at the cardiac catheter. A special device was applied to prevent the obstruction of the ventricular catheter. In spite of all endeavours, the already ample list of severe and frequent complications continued to increase just as the disillusionment from venous shunts. In current years peritoneal shunting has gained many advocates.

Again, after the first enthusiasm about the results achieved even with ventriculo-peritoneal sylastic catheters or with the new procedures of lumboperi-

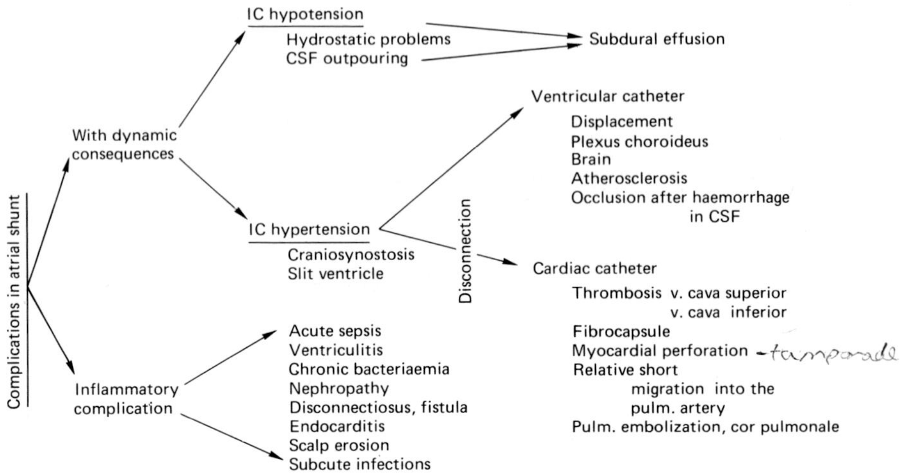

Fig. 1. Complications in atrial shunt.

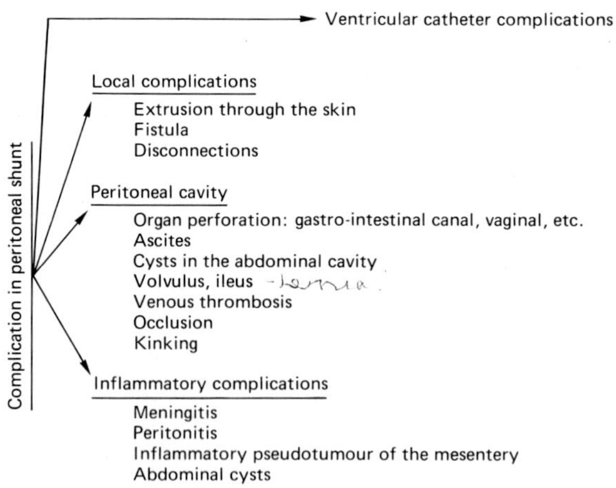

Fig. 2. Complication in peritoneal shunt.

toneal drainage, and recently with the one-piece shunts, a new impressive list, this time of the complications of peritoneal shunts has accumulated (fig. 2).

It is beyond doubt that: (1) the peritoneal shunts have eliminated septicaemia; (2) the grave complications have been replaced by milder though frequent peritoneal complications (hernia, volvulus, ileus, organ perforation etc.) whose late sequelae are not yet known.

I am in no way entitled to offer my opinion as to any preference in method, and I do not think it justified to do so only in the light of merely this list of complications. I only wish to summarize our practice accepted on the basis of our experience with 550 shunt implantations, from which 460 were infantile hydrocephalus cases.

(1) In the premature or new-born infant we prefer a peritoneal shunt because it means less stress for the patient, because of the narrow lumina of the cervical veins, and because the relative growth rate is the highest in this period. A peritoneal shunt is applied in infancy also when the patient's condition and, consequently, surgical tolerance are both poor. Finally, peritoneal shunt seems to be the most advisable also after bacterial meningitis and ventriculitis.

(2) An atrial shunt is employed in all other cases. It should be pointed out that the training and personal preference of the operating surgeon also influence the choice of procedure.

In conclusion, I think if the complications of the two most extensively used methods are weighed in the two scales of a balance, the pile would be quite impressive on either side. It is hard to tell which pile would be heavier. It is up to you to turn the scales in one direction.

Dr. E. Paraicz, National Institute of Neurosurgery, Budapest (Hungary)

Monogr. neural Sci., vol. 8, pp. 52–54 (Karger, Basel 1982)

Abdominal Complications of CSF-Peritoneal Shunts

Daniel S. Rush[a], *John W. Walsh*[b]

[a]Department of Surgery, [b]Division of Neurosurgery, University of Kentucky Medical Center, Lexington, Ky., USA

Intra-abdominal complications associated with cerebrospinal fluid (CSF)-peritoneal shunts are unusual. 40 abdominal complications developed in 38 of 300 consecutive patients with shunts at the University of Kentucky Medical Center, Lexington, Ky., from January 1, 1970, to December 31, 1979.

Clinical Material

The 300 patients in this series were all under 16 years of age. The initial CSF-peritoneal shunt was placed in 191 patients (64%) under 1 year of age, 55 patients (18%) between ages 2 and 7 years, and 54 patients (18%) after 8 years of age. 517 shunt procedures were performed on these patients with a mean of 1.7 shunt procedures per patient.

91% had a ventriculo-peritoneal shunt placed, 6% had a theco-peritoneal shunt and 3% had a subdural-peritoneal shunt. The Pudenz distal slit-valve cathether with a proximal reservoir was used most commonly until 1973 (17% of the total shunting procedures). The Raimondi spring-reinformed, distal slit-valve catheter was used between 1974 and 1975 (22%). The valveless Cordis distal catheter with a proximal Hakim valve has been used exclusively since 1976 (61%).

Abdominal Complications

General Considerations. The overall complication rate in this series was 13%. Abdominal complications were either septic in nature or resulted from a mechanical failure in the shunt catheter or from a disturbance of absorption of CSF by the peritoneum. Complications developed in 35% of the age group under 1 year (mostly inguinal hernias), 45% of the 2- to 7- year-old group and 20% of the 8- to 16- year-old age group. This data suggests that increased age alone does not contribute to the likelihood that an abdominal complication will occur.

Patients having nonseptic abdominal complications had the same mean number of shunt procedures, or less, as did the whole population (1.7 proce-

Table I. Incidence of intra-abdominal complications as related to preceding shunt placement or revision

Complications	Number	Mean age (months) at first shunting	Number of mean shunts	Mean age (months) at complication	Mean duration from shunt placement to complication
Catheter migration	4	42 (1–110)	1.75 (1–3)	54 (14–127)	10 (1–20)
Inguinal hernia	17	4 (1–29)	1.35 (1–3)	13 (1–55)	8 (1–30)
CSF ascites	4	52 (3–117)	1.75 (1–3)	55 (3–119)	1 (1–2)
CSF pseudocyst	4	30 (10–67)	1.75 (1–3)	62 (47–89)	19 (1–42)
Intra-abdominal sepsis	5	66 (1–152)	2 (1–4)	67 (4–153)	1 (1)
Perforated viscus	2	22 (20–24)	2.5 (2–3)	46 (25–66)	22 (1–42)

Table II. Relationship of catheter type to incidence of intra-abdominal complications.

Complications	Type of catheter			Total
	Pudenz	Raimondi	Cordis	
Catheter migration	0	4	0	4
Inguinal hernia	1	1	15	17
CSF ascites	1	1	2	4
CSF pseudocyst	0	1	3	4
	2	7	20	29
Intra-abdominal sepsis	1	3	1	5
Perforated viscus	0	2	0	2
	1	5	1	7[1]

[1] Excluding 2 cases of acute appendicitis, 1 case of intra-abdominal adhesion, and 2 cases of catheter migration occurring in the same patient.

dures per patient) as shown in table I. Likewise, none of the different catheters were associated with nonseptic complication more often than its use would predict (table II).

Septic complications, however, occurred in patients having a greater than average number of shunts than did the population as a whole (table I) and five of the seven septic complications occurred in patients with the Raimondi spring-reinforced catheter (table II). There has been a sharp decline in the number of shunt-related septic abdominal complications in the last 4 years.

There was one death in the series following a cardiorespiratory arrest in the postoperative period in a patient who had undergone correction of an incarcerated hydrocele.

Nonseptic Complications. Inguinal hernias occurred in 17 children (7% of the population under seven years of age). 6 children were born prematurely. 7 cases were bilateral inguinal hernias and 2 others were associated with umbilical hernias. 4 cases of communicating hydroceles resolved spontaneously. 1 case of an acute incarcerated hydrocele occurred and was followed by a cardiorespiratory arrest in the postoperative period unrelated to the operative procedure. Hernias and hydroceles, caused by increased intra-abdominal fluid pressure and failure of closure of the processus vaginalis, are more common in this population.

CSF ascites developed in 4 patients. 3 of these had recently undergone laparotomy unrelated to the shunting procedure. There were 4 cases of CSF pseudocyst. All of these patients had recently had shunt infections or active ventriculitis. Diagnosis was confirmed by abdominal X-ray, ultrasound and computer-assisted tomography. Complete resolution in all of these cases was obtained only after removal of the shunt catheter. CSF ascites and pseudocyst appear to be due to malabsorption of CSF by the peritoneum secondary to subclinical peritonitis.

No ill effects were seen in 4 children with disconnection of the shunt catheter from the proximal reservoir and migration of the shunt tubing into the abdominal cavity. The catheter was removed in only 2 cases. Kinking of the shunt catheter occurred in 1 patient and another patient had a migratory acute abdominal pain associated with the location of the catheter tip. Symptoms resolved following removal of the shunt catheter.

Septic Complications. 2 cases of intestinal perforation occurred in patients with the Raimondi spring-reinforced catheter. Both children presented with Gram-negative ventriculitis and an unremarkable abdominal examination. The catheter tip was protruding from the anus in 1 case. Resolution occurred following removal of the shunt and antibiotic therapy.

5 patients developed peritonitis or intra-abdominal abscesses. All of these had an active shunt infection and acute abdominal pain. These patients also recovered after administration of antibiotics and removal of their shunt.

2 patients developed acute abdominal pain from appendicitis. Neither has ventriculitis or shunt infection. Diagnosis in 1 case was facilitated by the demonstration of an appendicolith on abdominal X-ray.

D.S. Rush, MD, Department of Surgery, University of Kentucky, Medical Center, Lexington, KY 40536 (USA)

Monogr. neural Sci., vol. 8, pp. 55–56 (Karger, Basel 1982)

Intraperitoneal Pseudocyst: Mimicking Liver Disease

John P. Latchaw, Jr., Joseph F. Hahn

Department of Neurological Surgery, The Cleveland Clinic Foundation, Cleveland, Ohio, USA

A 40-year-old male presented to the Cleveland Clinic for evaluation of progressive abdominal discomfort. The patient recalled that the pain began 1 week prior to admission. The discomfort was characterized as a continuous dull ache confined to the upper abdomen unrelated to fatty foods. He denied flank or back pain. The patient denied any change in bowel habits or stool color. Nausea, vomiting, and urologic symptoms were absent. The patient denied a history of duodenal ulcer. The patient underwent a ventriculoperitoneal shunt for aqueductal stenosis, 1 month prior to admission.

Physical examination revealed a blood pressure of 120/80. Pulse rate was 80 and regular. There were no palpable masses and diffuse guarding was present. Maximal tenderness was found 4 cm inferolateral to the xiphoid in the right upper quadrant. Rebound and percussion tenderness were not present. Rectal examination was normal. The remainder of the physical examination was unremarkable.

Electrolytes, coagulation studies, lipase, urine amylase, and urinalysis were within normal limits. Hepatitis B surface antigen was negative. Total bilirubin, SGOT, and alkaline phosphatase were mildly elevated. SGPT, CPK, and GGTP were markedly increased. Multiple blood counts failed to demonstrate leukocytosis although a predominance of neutrophils (average 72%) was noted on differential examination.

Upright abdominal roentgenogram revealed paralytic ileus and a catheter tip overlying the liver. A small pleural effusion was observed on chest roentgenogram. Gallium scanning suggested a subdiaphragmatic abscess. Abdominal CAT scan demonstrated the intraperitoneal catheter and a right anterior suprahepatic hypodense area compatible with a pseudocyst.

In the operating theater, the distal catheter was withdrawn through a 2-cm abdominal incision and 300 ml of clear fluid immediately discharged from the incision. CSF cultures were negative. The distal tubing was repositioned and immediately reinserted into the right lower quadrant. Shunt and pseudocyst cultures were sterile. The patient's discomfort resolved and hepatic enzymes returned to normal. 6 months after operation, the patient returned with a shunt infection. The shunt was externalized and the patient was treated with antibiotics. After satisfactory recovery, the shunt was reinserted into the peritoneal cavity. The unique feature of our case is the elevated hepatic enzymes. We suspect that the pseudocyst which compressed the liver caused (1) intense right upper quadrant pain, (2) elevated enzymes indicative of liver dysfunction, and (3) localized pleural effusion.

Peritoneal pseudocyst secondary to shunt dysfunction is not a common problem. When it does occur, it is often related to shunt infection [1], previous abdominal operations [2], or CSF with high protein content [3]. None of these factors are always present. Our patient did not have elevated CSF protein, previous abdominal surgery or evidence of CSF infection at the time of diagnosis of pseudocyst. Infection appeared 6 months later. We believe this may have been a factor in causation of the pseudocyst but cannot explain why it was so indolent.

The abdominal CAT scan led to the diagnosis. We suggest that this study be done on all patients with abdominal complaints who have a peritoneal shunt.

Finally, the elevated liver enzymes are unique. To our knowledge, this problem has never been reported. The enzymes promptly cleared after the first surgery. We believe that localized pressure on the liver caused the elevation.

References

1 Parry, S.W.; Schumacher, J.F., Llewelyn, R.C.: Abdominal pseudocysts and ascities formation after ventriculoperitoneal shunt procedures. J. Neurosurg. *43:* 476–480 (1975).

2 DeSousa, A.L.; Worth, R.M.: Extrusion of peritoneal catheter through abdominal incision: report of a rare complication of ventriculoperitoneal shunt. Neurosurgery *5:* 504–505 (1979).

3 Davidson, R.I.; Lingely, J.F.: Intraperitoneal pseudocyst: treatment by aspiration. Surg. Neurol. *4:* 33–36 (1975).

J.P. Latchaw, MD, Department of Neurological Surgery, The Cleveland Clinic Foundation, Cleveland, OH (USA)

Mnogr. neural Sci., vol. 8, pp. 57–58 (Karger, Basel 1982)

Stress Fracture of Wire-Reinforced Shunt Tubing

J. Haase

Department of Neurosurgery, Odense University Hospital, Odense, Denmark

Disregarding the enormous amount of shunt procedures performed, very few reports deals with the bio-mechanical structure of shunt systems. In order to prevent kinking of peritoneal shunts, wire-reinforced Silastic tubing was introduced and has in our hands served its purpose.

However, recently 3 children suffered rupture of the tubing close to the plastic connectors (fig. 1). The assemble was placed behind the ear, and we suggest that the ruptures occurred because head-turning pulled the distal end of the tubing, thus causing severe stress at the end of the connectors. We know that longitudinal pulling may produce changes in wire-reinforced Silastic tubing which is demonstrated in figure 2. It is therefore a question whether the longitudinal stress changes the anti-kinking characteristics of the tubing, resulting in fractures.

To the best of our knowledge these fractures have not been reported. They emphasize the necessity for an international device standard for shunt valves and tubing.

For figures see reverse side.

J. Haase, MD, Department of Neurosurgery, Odense University Hospital, DK-5000 Odense (Denmark)

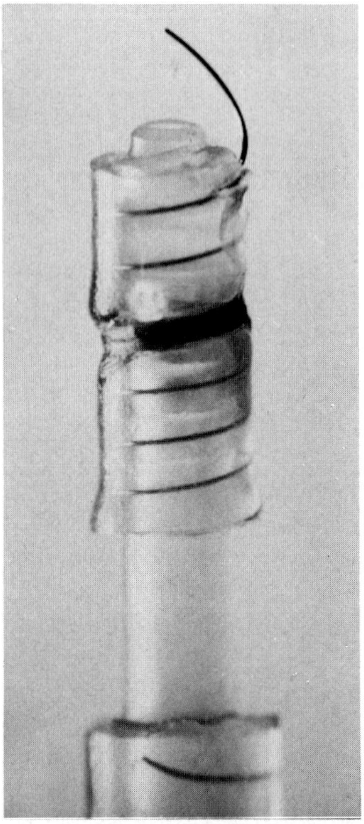

Fig. 1. Rupture of the tubing close to the plastic connectors.

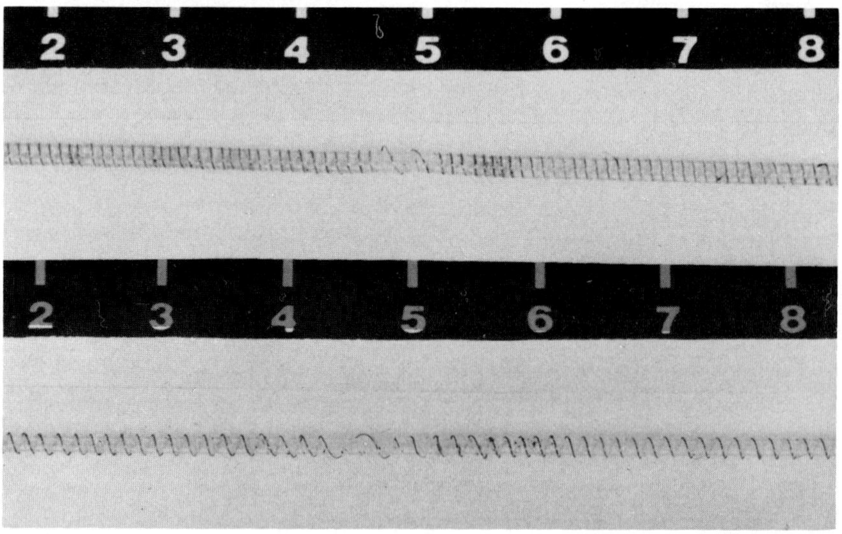

Fig. 2. Changes produced in Silastic tubing by longitudinal pulling.

Monogr. neural Sci., vol. 8, pp. 59–62 (Karger, Basel 1982)

Histological Study of the Obstructing Agents in Ventriculoperitoneal Shunts

Laligam N. Sekhar[a], *John Moossy*[b], *A.N. Guthkelch*[a]
[a]Department of Neurosurgery, [b]Department of Neuropathology,
University of Pittsburgh, Pittsburgh, Pa., USA

Malfunction due to obstruction is a significant problem associated with ventriculoperitoneal (VP) shunts. The pathology and shunt malfunction is however poorly defined. We are reporting in detail the gross and histological findings from a consecutive series of malfunctioning shunts.

Material and Methods

201 consecutive shunt revisions performed on 114 hydrocephalic patients over a period of 16 months at the Children's Hospital of Pittsburgh provided the material for this study. The revisions were prompted by clinical indications of shunt failure, along with computed tomographic confirmation in the majority of instances. All but five of the shunts revised consisted of Raimondi three-piece systems. The tissues inside and outside the malfunctional shunt catheters were examined and measured grossly and processed for histology. The sections were routinely stained with hematoxylin and eosin and special stains such as Gram stain and PTAH (phosphotungstic acid hematoxylin) were used when indicated.

Results

Malfunction of the shunt occurred in continuity in 163 instances. Disconnection was present in 18 and extraperitoneal migration in five. The ventricular end was obstructed in 73, the peritoneal end in 62 and both in 47 cases; no obstruction was found in 4 disconnection cases and in 15 other shunts. 90 ventricular ends and 50 peritoneal ends were submitted for pathological examination. Obstructive materials were found at the tips but not along the course of the shunt. On gross examination, whitish gray to yellowish brown material, sometimes discolored by hemorrhage, was often found at the ventricular end, always confined to the region of the holes (first 15 mm). At the peritoneal end, the

Table I. Histopathology of obstructing tissues

		Ventricular end (n = 91)	Peritoneal end (n = 50)
I	Tissures normal to region		
	Choroid plexus	35	–
	Glial tissues	36	–
	Connective tissue	49	33
	Leptomeninges	21	–
	Brain tissue	15	–
	Ependyma	15	–
	Mesothelial cells		17
II	Pathological tissues		
	Inflammation		
	Acute	13	17
	Chronic	45	28
	Granulomatous	44	23
	Necrosis	5	24
	Hemorrhage		
	Recent	10	3
	Old	17	7
	Fibrin	17	22
	Tumor	3	
	Calcium	6	7
III	Foreign material		
	Cotton	10	7
	Hair	5	4
	Talc	6	7
	Bacteria	3	1
	Unidentified	5	12
IV	Embolic tissue		
	Choroid plexus	–	4
	Leptomeninges	–	2
	Tumor	–	1
V	No luminal tissue	8	5

commonest finding was that of yellowish white material inside the tubing in the region of the slits. The histological findings are categorized (table I) under five major headings: tissues normally found in the region (although abnormally proliferated at times), pathological tissues, foreign bodies, embolized tissue, and no luminal tissue.

Discussion

Malfunction of shunts may be considered separately as ventricular end malfunction, peritoneal end malfunction and malfunction of connecting parts, including valves. At the *ventricular end,* choroid plexus has been popularly considered to be the most important obstructive tissue. *Hakim* [4] also found other materials such as brain tissue, connective tissue, protein, fibrin and leukocytes. *Collins et al.* [1] in a scanning electron microscopic study, correlated ventricular catheter position with pathology; choroid plexus was found more frequently inside catheter tips located behind the foramen of Monro and ependyma more frequently when the catheter tips were located in front [5]. Placement of the catheter tip in the choroid plexus free frontal horn has been correlated with prolonged shunt function for ventriculoatrial shunts [6]. However, once placed, migration of the catheter tip within the ventricular system may occur initially because of shrinkage of ventricles with resolution of hydrocephalus or later, because of normal head growth. In our material, not only choroid plexus and ependyma but also leptomeninges, glial tissue, connective tissue and brain tissue (subependymal astrocytes, neurons and white matter) were found.

Acute and chronic inflammatory changes were found frequently at both ends. Acute inflammation was seen in the absence of culture proven infection in 28 cases and this perhaps includes some cases of occult infection not culturable by routine methods, as pointed out by *Fokes* [2]. A randomized study of antibiotic prophylaxis has also suggested that indolent shunt infection may be an important cause of shunt malfunction [3].

A variety of foreign bodies was found imbedded in the tissues: cotton fibers, hair, talc granules, and unidentified foreign bodies. Their identification was facilitated by polarized light, they were usually surrounded by foreign body giant cells. *Hair* was presumably derived from the patient or operating room personnel and *cotton fibers* from cottonoids and sponges used during the operation. *Talc granules,* with a typical Maltese cross appearance, were seen with equal frequency at the ventricular and peritoneal ends. The talc was most likely derived from gloves.

Tumor cells were found in a patient with medulloblastoma and on two occasions in a patient with subependymal giant cell astrocytoma. The patient with medulloblastoma had positive cytology for cells in the cerebrospinal fluid and in the patient with the giant cell astrocytoma, the tip of the shunt was embedded in tumor.

Scant information exists in the literature about the pathology at the *peritoneal end.* In our study, 17 peritoneal ends demonstrated mesothelial cells peculiar to the peritoneal cavity. Connective tissue and inflammatory changes were as frequent as at the ventricular end but fibrin and necrotic changes were more frequent. The significance of foreign bodies has been commented upon previously. Embolization of not only tumor cells (giant cell astrocytoma) but also normal tissues (meninges and choroid plexus) was found. *Hoffman et al.* [5] have pointed out the possibility of shunt embolization in medulloblastoma metastases. In addition, embolization of normal tissues may occasionally contribute to peritoneal end malfunction. Obstruction of the shunt with surface film only ('no luminal tissue') seemed to occur with equal frequency at both ends. However, since the proportion of obstructed peritoneal catheters submitted was smaller than the ventricular, this observation may be incorrect.

Conclusion

In addition to the importance of ventricular catheter position and inflammation, our studies suggest the possible role of foreign body contamination and shunt embolization of tissues in shunt malfunction.

References

1 Collins, P.; Hockley, A.D.; Woollam, D.H.M.: Surface ultrastructure of tissues occluding ventricular catheters. J. Neurosurg. *48:* 609–613 (1973).

2 Fokes, E.C.: Occult infections of ventriculoatrial shunts. J. Neurosurg. *33:* 517–622 (1970).

3 Haines, S.J.; Taylor, F.: Prophylactic methicillin for shunt operations: effects on incidence of shunt malfunction and infection. Presented at the Annual Meeting by the Pediatric section of the American Association of Neurological Surgeons, December 1980, New York.

4 Hakim, S.: Observations on the physiopathology of the CSF pulse and prevention of ventricular catheter obstruction in valve shunts. Devl Med. Child Neurol. *11:* suppl., pp. 42–48 (1969).

5 Hoffman, H.J.; Hendrick, E.B.; Humphreys, R.P.: Metastasis via ventriculoperitoneal shunt in patients with medulloblastoma. J. Neurosurg. *44:* 562–566 (1976).

6 Illingworth, R.D.; Logue, V.; Symon, L.; Uemura, K.: The ventriculocaval shunt in the treatment of adult hydrocephalics. Results and complications in 101 patients. J. Neurosurg. *35:* 681–685 (1971).

L.N. Sekhar, MD, Department of Neurosurgery, University of Pittsburgh, Pittsburgh, PA 15213 (USA)

Monogr. neural Sci., vol. 8, pp. 63–65 (Karger, Basel 1982)

Histological Response to Ventricular Catheters

A.D. Hockley

The Queen Elizabeth Hospital, Edgbaston, Birmingham, England

The problem of ventricular catheter obstruction in hydrocephalus was studied by scanning electron microscopy of the tissue within occluded catheters from 16 patients, and histological examination of cerebral tissue at post-mortem from 3 patients at varying intervals of time after catheter insertion.

As previously reported [1], 16 occluded ventricular catheters were removed at the time of shunt revision and in 10 specimens, choroid plexus, with each cell surface showing microvilli and cilia, was found. Ependymal tissue was observed in 5 specimens. In addition to fibrin clots, capillary formation was seen frequently, suggesting active growth of the occluding tissue. Appearances were correlated with the position and length of time the catheter was in place, confirming the observation that catheters posterior to the foramen of Monro are more likely to be occluded by choroid plexus, and anterior catheters by ependyma. The quantity of tissue did not bear any relationship to the duration of insertion. Of the occluded catheters, 7 were placed anterior and 9 posterior to the foramen of Monro.

In 3 necropsy specimens, 8 days, 2 months and 1 year after catheter insertion, macroscopic examination of the brain revealed a clearly demarcated channel extending through white matter to ventricle (fig. 1). In the first case, a ventricular catheter had been used for intraventricular administration of antibiotics in a patient with severe meningitis. Histologically, the white matter showed scattered pericapillary haemorrhages and myelin pallor due to oedema. Swollen terminals of disrupted adjacent neurones were seen, but at this stage little in the way of astrocytic response (fig. 2). In the other cases, a ventriculo-atrial shunt had been inserted for obstructive hydrocephalus, and a more established cell response was seen. The microglia in contact with the catheter had fused to form multinucleate foreign body type giant cells, and these flattened cells in places formed an almost continuous lining (fig. 3). In addition to many swollen axon terminals, hypertrophied reactive astrocytes produced a glial fibrous network to wall off the

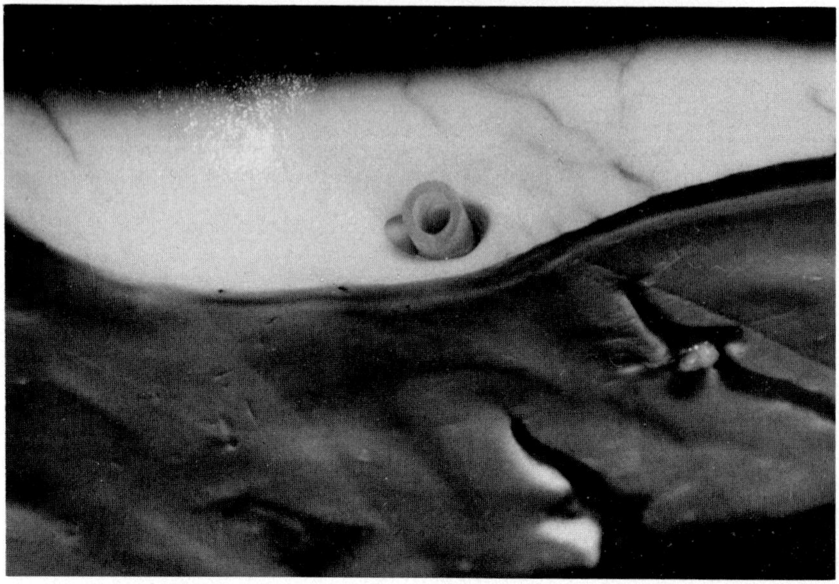

Fig. 1. Coronal section of brain showing catheter protruding through wall of ventricle. × 3.2

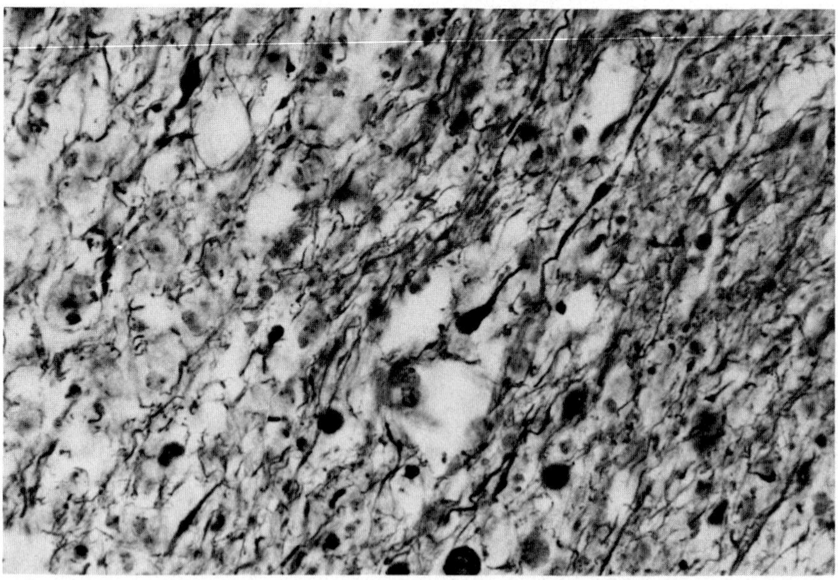

Fig. 2. Disruption of axons with swollen terminals along catheter path. Palmgren's silver stain. × 240.

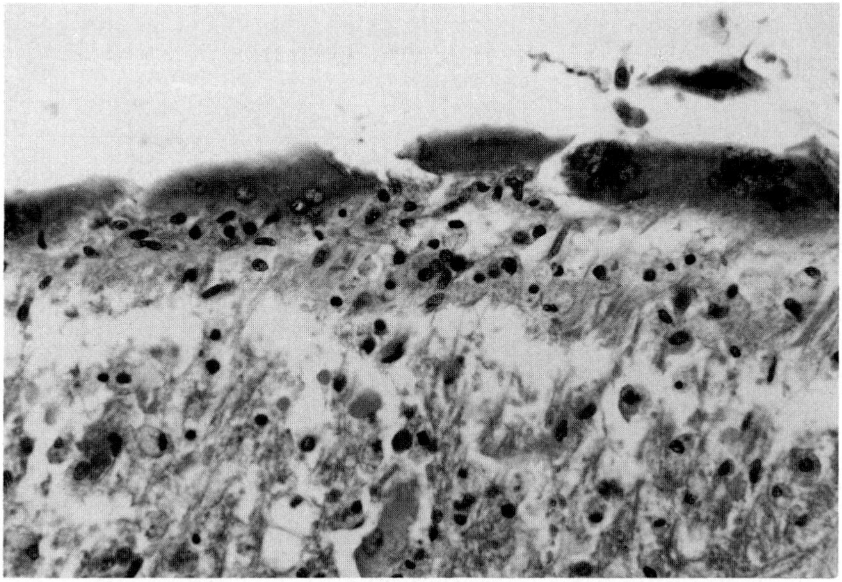

Fig. 3. Catheter channel lined by multinucleate giant cells. Haematoxylin and eosin. × 240.

catheter track, but there were no obvious changes on the ventricular surface. Finally, in the third case, the cellular response was largely replaced by fibrous gliosis. The very clearly defined narrow channel through cerebral tissue and the scanty haemosiderin deposition indicate that, once inserted, there is virtually no movement of the catheter from its original position.

From this small series with a similar incidence of catheter obstruction for anteriorly and posteriorly placed catheters, there would seem to be no optimum site for ventricular catheter insertion, and it has become the author's practice to use the most dilated part of the ventricle as shown by CT scan.

References

Collins, P.; Hockley, A.D.; Woollam, D.H.M.: Surface ultrastructure of tissues occluding ventricular catheters. J. Neurosurg. *48:* 609–613 (1978).

A.D. Hockley, FRCS, The Queen Elizabeth Hospital, Edgbaston, Birmingham B15 2TH England)

Monogr. neural Sci., vol. 8, pp. 66–68 (Karger, Basel 1982)

Infection Rate with and without Prophylactic Antibiotic Therapy after Shunt Insertion for Hydrocephalus

José A. Alvarez-Garijo, Manuel Vila Mengual
Pediatric Neurosurgery Unit, Hospital Infantil 'La Fé', Valencia, Spain

Infection rate after shunt insertion for hydrocephalus shows figures ranging from 5 to 34% according to different diagnosis criteria [2, 5, 6]. It is widely accepted that the infection usually has a surgical origin [1, 3, 4]. Routine prophylactic antibiotic therapy is generally used although its usefulness was not definitively stated. This study was carried out upon 163 patients with hydrocephalus, aged 1 month to 6 years and separated in two groups according to respective treatment.

The 90 patients of group I were treated by ventriculoperitoneal shunt system composed by a Raimondi peritoneal spring catheter and a Pudenz ventricular catheter with pump reservoir. Systemic antibiotic therapy was given during the postoperative period in all cases and also before the operation in 12 patients in which previous infection was detected or suspected by clinical data with or without bacteriological confirmation. This preoperative treatment was stopped when the cure was achieved as clinical and laboratory data demonstrated and 9 of these infected patients underwent surgery immediately while the other 3 were operated on a few weeks later, but without pre-operative CSF or blood culture.

The 73 patients of group II were treated by ventriculoperitoneal shunt system composed by a Raimondi peritoneal spring catheter and a Salmon-Rickham ventriculostomy reservoir. During the postoperative period no systemic antibiotic was given and ventricular CSF cultures were done every 2 days. 10 patients with preoperative infection were treated by antimicrobial agents (locally when it was feasible) until clinical and laboratory data demonstrated total cure and surgery was done only when repeated cultures, without treatment, were negative and never before 15 days after the antimicrobial treatment was stopped.

The study was carried out in non-contemporary groups, but all patients were treated by the same surgical team and the same procedures including per-

Table I. Shunt infections in 90 patients (group I)

Case	Previous infection	Antibiotic	Infection	Organism
1	no	methicillin	ventriculitis	Pseudomona
2	no	methicillin	ventriculitis	*S. aureus*
3	no	methicillin	ventriculitis	*S. epidermidis*
4	no	methicillin	ventriculitis	*S. epidermidis*
5	no	methicillin	ventriculitis	Pseudomona
6	ventriculitis *H. influenzae*	methicillin	ventriculitis	*H. influenzae*
7	no	methicillin	ventriculitis	Pseudomona
8	no	methicillin	ventriculitis	*S. aureus*
9	sepsis *E. coli*	methicillin gentamicin	ventriculitis	*E. coli*
10	no	methicillin gentamicin	ventriculitis	*S. epidermidis*
11	sepsis *E. coli*	methicillin	ventriculitis	*E. coli*
12	no	methicillin	ventriculitis	*S. epidermidis*
13	sepsis unidentified organism	methicillin	ventriculitis	*S. aureus*
14	no	methicillin	ventriculitis	Pseudomona
15	no	methicillin gentamicin	ventriculitis	*S. epidermidis*
16	no	methicillin	ventriculitis	*S. epidermidis*

operative irrigation of the surgical field and shunt elements with antibiotic serum saline solution.

In group I, during a follow-up of 28–44 months, 16 patients (17%) became infected, 4 of them belonging to the previous infected subgroup. In these 4 patients the causal organism was the same as in the first infection (table I).

In group II, during a follow-up of 8–17 months, only 1 infection was detected (1.3%) and this occurred in a patient with previous infection (table II).

These results call our attention to two facts: (1) the influence of preoperative infection and its management in the postoperative infection rate, and (2) the negative effect of prophylactic antibiotic therapy. A possible partial explanation for this striking fact may be the ability of some organisms, including normally non-pathogenic organims, such as *Staphylococcus epidermidis,* to become resistant under antibiotic therapy. We have found no data about the role of the loss of normal balance between the different bacteria.

Table II. Infection rate after shunt insertion

	Patients	Infected (%)
Group I (with antibiotic therapy)		
With previous infection	12	4 (33)
Without previous infection	78	12 (15)
Total	90	16 (17)
Group II (without antibiotic therapy)		
With previous infection	10	1 (10)
Without previous infection	63	0 –
Total	73	1 (1.3)

We have used a ventriculostomy reservoir to avoid routine antibiotic therapy. This allows us an accurate infection control by means of seriated CSF cultures. In fact, the only infection in group II was detected by CSF culture, before the symptoms started, and was successfully treated by the intraventricular way using the same reservoir, saving the ventriculoperitoneal shunt.

Our results suggest the importance of an accurate control of previous infection, the uselessness of prophylactic antimicrobial agents, and support our proposed management using a ventriculostomy reservoir.

References

1 Bayston, R.; Spitz, L.: The role of retrograde movement of bacteria in ventriculo-atrial shunt colonisation. Z. Kinderchir. *25:* 352–356 (1978).

2 Guidetti, B.; Guiffré, R.; Palma, L.; Fontana, M.: Hydrocephalus in infancy and childhood. Our experience in CSF shunting. Child's Brain *2:* 209–225 (1976).

3 Keucher, T.R.; Mealey, J.: Long-term results after ventriculoatrial and ventriculoperitoneal shunting for infantile hydrocephalus. J. Neurosurg. *50:* 179–186 (1979).

4 Luthardt, T.: Bacterial infections in ventriculo-auricular shunt systems. Devl Med. Child Neurol. *22:* suppl., pp. 105–109 (1970).

5 Raimondi, A.J.; Robinson, J.S.; Kuwamura, K.: Complications of ventriculoperitoneal shunting and a critical comparison of the three-piece and one-piece systems. Child's Brain *3:* 321–342 (1977).

6 Scarff, T.B.; Nelson, P.B.; Reigel, H.D.: External drainage for ventricular infection following cerebrospinal fluid shunts. Child's Brain *4:* 129–136 (1978).

Dr. J.A. Alvarez-Garijo, Neurocirugia Pediátrica. Hospital Infantil 'La Fé', Avda Campanar, 21, Valencia (Spain)

Monogr. neural Sci., vol. 8, pp. 69–71 (Karger, Basel 1982)

Shunt Infections: A Protocol for Effective Treatment

Kenneth Shapiro, Kenneth Shulman
Albert Einstein College of Medicine, Bronx, N.Y., USA

A variety of medical and surgical strategies have been proposed for the treatment of children with infected shunts [1–3]. Although all methods are useful in some patients, it is our belief that treatment of the infected shunt should be expeditious in order to avoid prolonged hospitalization and secondary complications. Since most of the strategies published by others have been employed at our institution, we have reviewed our experience in 43 consecutive cases of pediatric shunt infection in order to develop an efficient, systematic approach to treating these children. The treatment algorithm outlined in figure 1 is our sequential approach to the infected shunt; the following discussion outlines how our experience led to this algorithm.

The cornerstone of all successful treatment is systemic and intraventricular antibiotics. The selection of antibiotics is based on in vitro disc sensitivity tests and the clinical response. However, the decision to treat with antibiotics alone or employ one of the surgical strategies is based on the time after the previous surgical procedure. During our review we found that only early infections were cured by medical management alone. Patients with infections becoming clinically manifest less than 60 days after the previous shunt manipulation are treated only by systemic and intraventricular antibiotics regardless of the infecting organism. However, we found that regardless of when the infection occurred, it was most appropriate to externalize all shunts associated with distal complications (peritonitis, wound infection, obstruction), other than bacteriemia. These distal complications occurred in 34% of our patients.

The next critical juncture in the treatment of the infected shunt is 6 days after initiating therapy. By then all patients in our series of successful treatment have shown clinical and laboratory signs of sterilization of the CSF and inferentially, the shunt. The patient is now euthermic, feeding normally and no longer irritable. We have found that this correlates well with sterile CSF. The CSF formula (protein, glucose, and cell counts) was totally unreliable in docu-

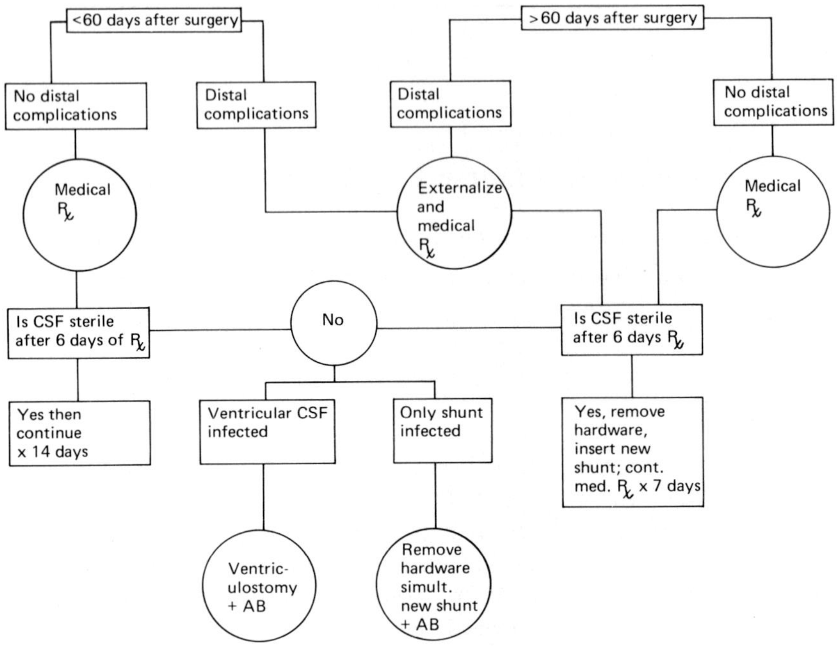

Fig. 1. Treatment algorithm used to treat the infected pediatric shunt.

menting the response of the infection to antibiotic therapy. In fact, CSF pleocytosis and hypoglycorrhachia may persist for weeks after sterilizing the CSF and shunt.

If the CSF is sterile after 6 days of treatment in patients who are to be treated medically, antibiotics are continued for approximately 2 weeks. Following this, several days should pass, and culture of CSF should be repeated off antibiotics. If the CSF is not sterile, one should then decide whether the infection resides only in the shunt hardware of whether the ventricular CSF is infected. If the ventricular CSF is infected in addition to the shunt being colonized, the shunt system should be removed and a separate clean ventriculostomy performed; treatment is begun again until the CSF is sterilized. If only the shunt is infected and the ventricular fluid is sterile, then the patient should undergo removal of all hardware and have simultaneous insertion of a new shunt on the contralateral side. Antibiotics should be continued for at least a week after inserting the new shunt.

Finally, we come to the group of patients treated with externalization whose CSF is sterile at 6 days or those treated by antibiotics but whose infection occurred more than 60 days after the last procedure. It is our belief that, regardless of whether these infections occurred early or late, the shunt apparatus should be removed and a new shunt inserted. When we have removed shunts in patients who have either been externalized or have had medical therapy alone and this has occurred more than 60 days after their previous surgery, the same organism has been cultured from the shunt as was originally cultured from the CSF in 20 of 22 patients. We interpret this finding as evidence of persistent colonization of the shunt. In our view, these infections are destined to recur.

Unlike others, we have evidence to support the treatment of infected shunts by antibiotics alone. Although we agree with *McLaurin* [1] that some functioning but infected shunts can be preserved if antibiotics are delivered directly to the CSF as well as systemically; we have found that not all shunt infections should be treated this way. We have tried to identify likely responders to a medical regime in order to minimize operative risks. Our study leads us to conclude that the early infections are most likely to respond to true medical management.

Using this algorithm for treating the infected shunt, we have been able to effectively treat and discharge most patients within 3 weeks after diagnosing a shunt infection. To us, this is the goal of treatment in infected pediatric shunts: rapid and effective therapy without prolonged hospitalization.

References

1 McLaurin, R.E.: Infected cerebrospinal fluid shunts. Surg. Neurol. *1:* 191–195 (1973).
2 Mori, K.; Raimondi, J.: An analysis of external ventricular drainage as a treatment for infected shunts. Child's Brain *1:* 243–250 (1975).
3 Nicholas, J.L.; Kamal, I.M.; Eckstein, H.B.: Immediate shunt replacement in the treatment of bacterial colonisation of Holter valves. Devl Med. Child Neurol. 22: suppl. *22:* 110–113 (1970).

K. Shapiro, MD, Albert Einstein College of Medicine, Bronx, NY (USA)

Monogr. neural Sci., vol. 8, pp. 72–74 (Karger, Basel 1982)

Shunt Infections in Hydrocephalic Children

A Retrospective and Prospective Study

M. Schepens, J. Berney

Paediatric and Neurosurgical Clinics, Geneva University Hospital, Geneva, Switzerland

In a first period no systematic bacteriological control was made at the time of an operation, either for insertion or for revision of a shunt. In a second period, samples of the CSF, the blood and portions of the shunting device were sent for bacteriological study. In a third period bacteriological examination of the 'steri-drape' covering the skin and of the wound swabs was added to the previous controls. This paper is a report on the observations made in reviewing the cases of non-tumoral hydrocephalus. All cases operated are used, except those lost to control or with a follow-up period of less than 18 months.

63 cases are available, concerning 57 ventriculo-atrial (VA, Holter) and 34 ventriculoperitoneal (VP, Ames) shunts. Prophylactic antibiotherapy was never used. 40 cases have never been treated for an infection of the shunt, but in 5 of them an *occult infection* could be detected in portions of the VA shunt. No treatment was given however and the children did well, because the contaminated system was in any case planned to be removed. The germ was always *Staphylococcus epidermidis.*

23 cases had to be treated for 29 clinical infections. These patients tend to be younger at the insertion of the valve than the non-infected ones (average age: 13.6 and 24.8 months). The number of revisions does not appear to be a very important factor in respect to infection, even if the number of operations for each child is almost double in the infected group (4.65) than in the non-infected group (2.6).

The 63 children were grouped as follows: not treated, 40; treated for infection, 23; contaminated, not treated, 5; not contaminated, 35. Infections treated, 29; occult infections, 8; external infections, 7; total number of internal contaminations, 30. Number of VA (Holter) shunts, 57; number of VP (Ames) shunts, 34; number of operations, 211. VA operations, 149, 149/57 = 2.6 operations/child, VP operations, 62, 62/34 = 1.8 operations/child (difference not significant). Number of operations for one treated child, 107/23 = 4.65. Number of operations for one non-treated child, 104/40 = 2.6 (the difference is significant).

7 infections are clearly related to surgical problems or mistakes, 3 due to *Staphylococcus aureus* and 4 to *Staph. epidermidis.* In these 7 cases pus was present or the tissues around the valve were infected. They are *external infections* and are similar to the usual wound infections. This type of infection has a frequency of 3.3% (7/211 operations). The other 22 infections are called *internal infections* and are all due to *Staph. epidermidis.* They are divided into 9 early infections, when the delay was less than 8 months (delay < 8 months; 50% < 3 months) and 13 *late infections,* with a longer delay (delay > 8 months; 50% > 20 months). To these 22 clinical infections must be added 5 occult infections in the non-treated groups and 3 occult infections in the infected group (2 VP and 1 VA). The total number of internal contaminations is 30.

The patent *internal infections* were about five times more frequent in VA than in VP shunts. This difference is very significant, but the risk for an infection to be treated after one operation is not significantly different in VA than in VP shunts, even if it is however four times higher in VA. If the total number of positive cultures for *Staph. epidermidis,* adding occult infections to treated infections, is compared in VA and VP, the difference is significant either in comparing them to the number of cases or to the number of operations. The apparent influence of the number of operations is due to the fact that in VA shunts revisions are more frequent. Number of children with not infected VA, 35; number of operations, 81 (2.31 operations/ child). Number of children with infected VA, 22; number of operations, 68 (3.1 operations/child; the difference is not significant). Number of VP operations, 62; number of VP internal contaminations, 4; risk of internal contaminations in VP operations, 4/62 = 0.065. Number of VA operations, 149; number of VA internal contaminations, 26; risk of internal contamination in VA shunt, 26/149 = 0.17. The risk of internal contamination is significantly higher with VA than with VP shunts.

In all the cases of clinical infection, the shunting material was, of course, contaminated (27 positive controls, but one negative, probably due to antibiotherapy). In VA shunt the blood can be either positive or negative, as it is in occult infections, with positive material. In most cases the new ventricular fluid was sterile (17 instances), but was contaminated in 4. The CSF taken from the valve was positive 10 times, but sterile 14 times, when the fluid was taken from the ventricular catheter, above the reservoir. Bacteriological controls of the operative field were more frequently positive in cases without infection and no correlation could be found between these results and subsequent occurrence of internal infection. Infection inside the device can last several months before it becomes clinically patent, since occult infection could retrospectively be traced in 7 cases, up to more than 6 months earlier in 3 cases.

The treatment was always successful, combining antibiotherapy (usually Cloxacillin) and removal of the infected material. Immediate replacement by a new shunt was successful in 5 instances, but in 6 cases it was not and external drainage was used. External drainage was always successful. 1 patient died of an unrelated cause.

M. Schepens, MD, Paediatric and Neurosurgical Clinics, Geneva University Hosptial, CH–1200 Geneva (Switzerland)

Monogr. neural Sci., vol. 8, pp. 75–77 (Karger, Basel 1982)

Management of Cerebrospinal Fluid Shunt Infections
A Clinical Experience

H.E. James[a] *J.W. Walsh*[c], *H.D. Wilson*[d] *J.D. Connor*[a,b]

[a]Division of Neurosurgery and [a,b]Department of Pediatrics, University of California at San Diego, Calif.; [c]Division of Neurosurgery and [d]Department of Pediatrics, University of Kentucky Medical Center, Lexington, Ky., USA

Introduction

There are currently three methods of treatment for the management of cerebrospinal fluid (CSF) shunt infections. All employ a combination of intravenous and intraventricular antibiotics, due to the unpredictable concentration of some antibiotics in ventricular fluid. In one method the shunt assembly is not removed and the antibiotic is administered through the shunt until the infection is cleared, supported with systemic antibiotics for a minimal period of 3 weeks [3, 6, 10]. A second method consists of removal of the existing shunt and during the same procedure insertion of a new shunt, followed by intrashunt antibiotic therapy as well as intravenous antibiotic therapy until the infection has resolved [2, 5]. Some authors have reported that the shunt assembly should be removed, external ventricular drainage instituted or a reservoir installed, and systemic and intraventricular antibiotics administered for a minimum period of 7 days. When the infection has been documented to be resolved, a new shunt may then be inserted [6–8].

This report deals with our experience with the three methods of treatment.

Materials and Methods

The patients were treated in the period from September 1975 to May 1980. Infection was documented by identification of bacterial organisms on culture of CSF obtained from the shunt. 36 patients also had simultaneous cultures of blood and urine as part of their preliminary evaluation.

Intravenous antibiotic therapy was started pending identification of the organism antibiotic susceptibility. When these results were available, the most appropriate antibiotic was instituted and definitive therapy begun. In 17 patients the shunt was removed and external ventricular drainage (EVD) instituted with twice daily antibiotic doses administered through the EVD (6 patients). In the remaining 11 patients no EVD was placed, but intermittent, once daily, ventricular punctures to the anterior fontanel were performed for decompression and antibiotic administration. In each case a total of 7 days of intraventricular and intravenous antibiotic therapy was administered. 13 patients underwent shunt removal with insertion of a new shunt during the same procedure, following 1 or 2 days of intravenous antibiotic therapy. The remaining 11 patients did not have their shunt removed. For both of these groups antibiotics were given twice daily through the shunt reservoir for a minimum period of 2 weeks, and by the intravenous route for 3 weeks. The concentration of antibiotics and ventricular fluid was measured at frequent intervals and the doses of medication adjusted to achieve optimal therapeutic concentrations. The antibiotic determinations were made by the method of *Simon et al.* [9] or of *Braude et al.* [1]. The intraventricular antibiotics employed were cephalothin, methicillin, nafcillin, ampicillin, gentamycin, in dosage ranges from 0.5 to 3.5 mg/kg/dose. The intravenous antibiotic administration was following the standard pediatric practice in reference to dosages employed for the therapy of meningitis.

48 h following completion of therapy all patients had ventricular CSF aspirations for cultures, as well as blood and urine cultures. A second CSF culture was obtained from all patients within 4 months after termination of therapy. An infection was said to be cured when both these CSF cultures were negative. The follow-up time ranged from 1 to 56 months, with a mean of 19 ± 12 months.

Results

There were 41 patients in the study with ages ranging from 2 months to 9 years. 5 patients had spina bifida, which had been repaired at birth. There were 31 ventriculoperitoneal shunts, one ventriculojugular shunt, one lumboperitoneal shunt; and 8 patients had two intracranial catheters connected to a single tube to the peritoneum. 36 patients had single organism infections and, as in other studies, the majority were due to Staphylococcus organisms. 5 patients had more than one infecting organism. There were 22 *Staphylococcus epidermidis* caused infections and five *Staphylococcus aureus.*

The 16 of 17 patients who had their shunts removed and either EVD or intermittent ventricular punctures were cured. In the group with shunt removal and immediate replacement there were 11 cures and 2 failures. Finally in the group in which the shunt was not removed, there were 4 successful results of the 11 patients treated (table I). 3 mortalities occurred, 2 of these in the group without shunt removals; 1 patient developed a more virulent and antibiotic-resistent superinfection and another patient expired when he was undergoing a very prolonged EVD therapy course. The third patient that expired belonged to the first treatment group, he consistently grew organisms during his intermittent ventricular punctures during therapy after the shunt was removed. He was a premature child with intracranial hemorrhage and an intracerebral infected hematoma that failed to sterilize with treatment.

Table I. Therapy and results in CSF infected shunts

	Number of patients	Successful trials	Unsuccessful trials	Mortality
With removal of shunt[1]	17	16	1	1
With removal and immediate replacement	13	11	2	0
Without removal of shunt	11	4	7	2

[1] Includes 1 patient who received intravenous antibiotics only (lumboperitoneal shunt).

References

1 Braude, A.I.; Bannister, J.; Wright, N.: Use of the gradient plate for routine clinical determinations of bacterial sensitivities to antibiotics. Antibiot. Annls *1954–1955:* 1133–1140.

2 Luckhardt, T.: Bacterial infections in ventriculo-auricular shunt systems. Devl Med. Child Neurol. *22:* suppl., pp. 105–109 (1970).

3 McLaurin, R.L.: Infected cerebrospinal fluid shunts. Surg. Neurol. *1:* 191–195 (1973).

4 O'Brien, M.; Parent, T.; Davis, B.: Management of ventricular shunt infections. Child's Brain *5:* 304–309 (1979).

5 Perrin, J.E.; McLaurin, F.L.: Infected ventriculo-atrial shunts. A method of treatment. J. Neurosurg. *27:* 21–26 (1967).

6 Sayers, M.P.: Shunt complications. Clin. Neurosurg. *23:* 393–400 (1976).

7 Schoenbaum, S.D.; Gardner, P.; Shillito, J.: Infections of cerebrospinal fluid shunts: epidemiology, clinical manifestations and therapy. J. infect. Dis. *131:* 543–552 (1975).

8 Shurtleff, D.B.; Christie, D.; Foltz, E.L.: Ventriculo-auriculostomy associated infection: a 12-year study. J. Neurosurg. *35:* 686–694 (1971).

9 Simon, H.J.; Yin, E.J.: Microbioassay of antimicrobial agents. Appl. Microbiol. *19:* 573–579 (1973).

10 Wald, S.L.; McLaurin, R.L.: Cerebrospinal fluid antibiotic levels during treatment of shunt infections. J. Neurosurg. *52:* 41–46 (1980).

H.E. James, MD, Division of Neurosurgery, University of California at San Diego, San Diego, CA 92103 (USA)

Monogr. neural Sci., vol. 8, pp. 78–80 (Karger, Basel 1982)

Calcified Subdural Empyema Post Ventriculoperitoneal Shunt for Hydrocephaly
Case Report

G.E. Ouaknine, R. Tadmor
Tel-Hashomer Hospital, Tel Aviv University, Tel Aviv, Israel

Subdural calcifications occurring in infancy and childhood are seldom reported in the literature. They are generally the late consequence of a traumatic subdural hematoma. A few cases of calcifications of post-meningitis subdural effusion are also reported. Occurrence of subdural hematoma is a well-known complication of shunt derivation for hydrocephaly but secondary calcification seems exceptional.

We present a case of calcified subdural empyema that occurred 8 years after a ventriculoperitoneal shunt for hydrocephaly.

Case Report

An 8-year-old child was admitted at the hospital because the parents – of primitive origin – could not bear any more the nauseous odor due to a 2 weeks continous flow of pus from the child's head.

On examination, the child was in fairly good condition without temperature, mildly retarded. After removing a lot of nauseous clothes around her head, one could see an enlarged head with a skin defect on the right parietal region, from where pus was flowing when tilting the head (fig. 1).

On skull X-rays, there was an enlargement of the head with diffuse thickening of the calvaria and a bilateral ovoid-shaped calcification, larger on the right side (fig. 2). A right carotid arteriography showed a right avascular zone corresponding to the calcified cavity with arteries in the midline and the cortical veins displaced medially by the mass (fig. 3). At the age of 4 months, the child was operated with a ventriculoperitoneal

Fig. 2. On the lateral film, there is an air fluid level with Foley catheter inserted within the calcified cavity for constant drainage and a skull defect corresponding to the previous burr hole for shunt (small black arrow). Small white arrows outline the cranial aperture surrounded by osteitis. The big black arrow shows the midline congenital defect.

1
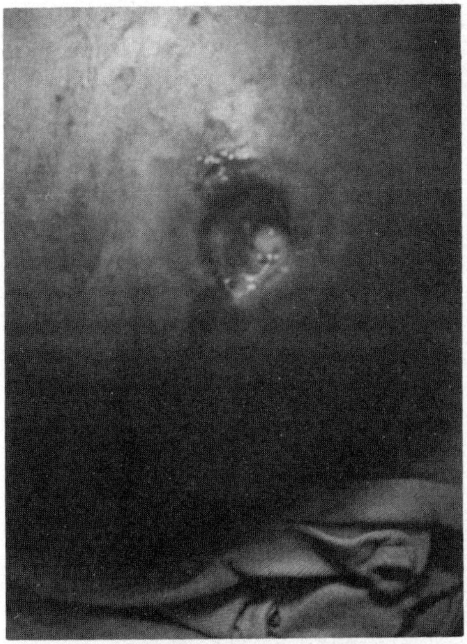

Fig. 1. After having shaved the scalp, one can see a skin defect on the right parietal region from where pus is flowing.

2
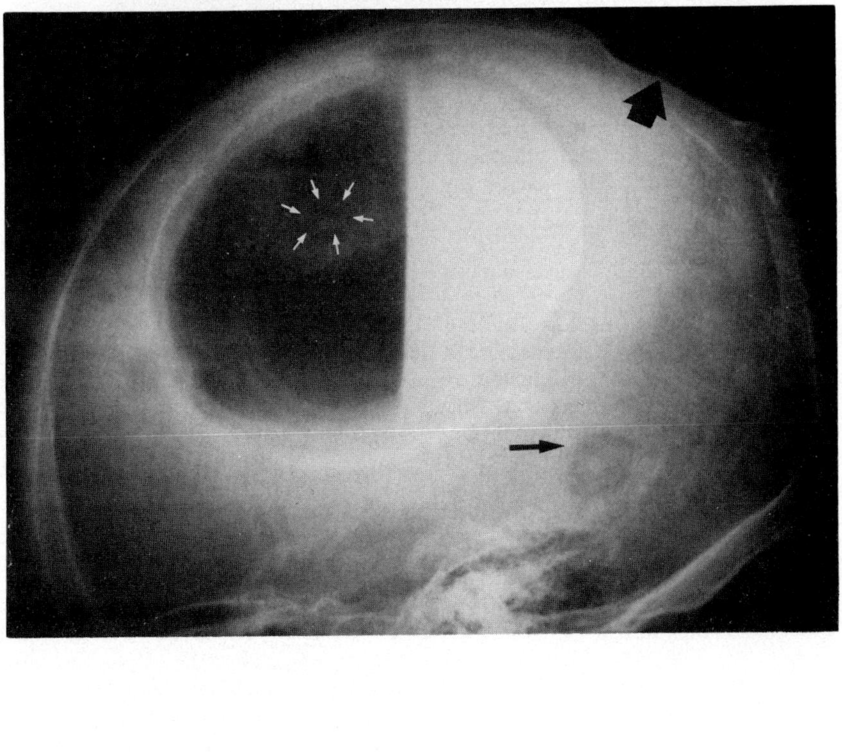

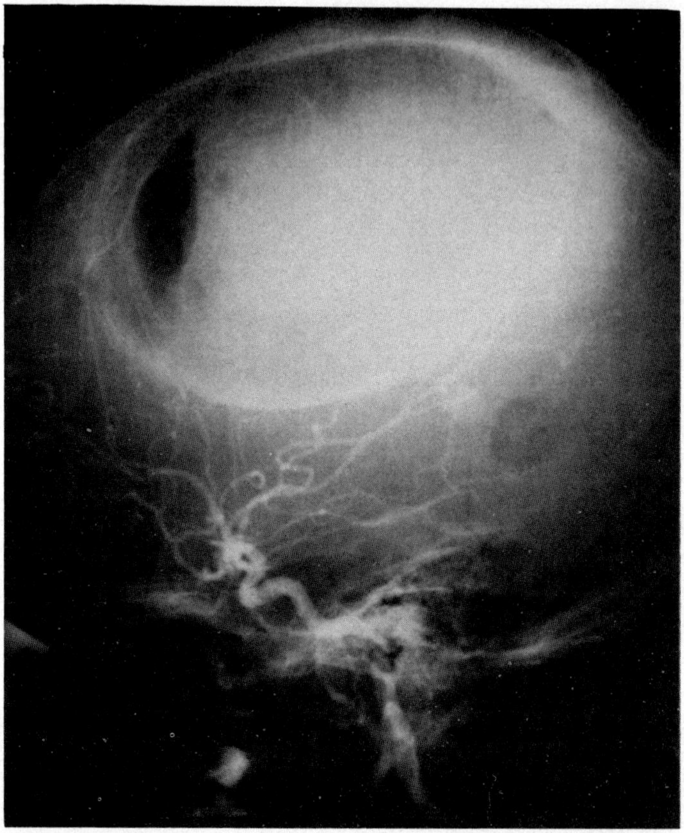

Fig. 3. Right carotid arteriography. On the lateral series, there is an avascular zone corresponding to the calcified cavity with splaying of the arteries.

shunt for hydrocephaly (medium pressure valve without antisiphon device). On examination, the shunt was not functioning any more.

The patient was explored and 160 ml of pus was removed through the hole, due most probably to the pressure sore of the scalp and local osteitis. The right encysted empyema was treated by continuous perfusion of antibiotics and drainage during several days until complete cleaning of the cavity. No attempt was made to remove the calcified mass. The pus remained sterile on different cultures. After plastic repair of the wound, the child was discharged in good condition and followed during 2 years without further complications.

G.E. Ouaknine, MD, Service of Neurosurgery, Notre-Dame Hospital,
1560 East Sherbrooke Street, Montreal, Que. H2L 4K8 (Canada)

Monogr. neural Sci., vol. 8, pp. 81–85 (Karger, Basel 1982)

Experimental and Clinical Studies on Pathogenesis of Intraventricular Septations following Meningoventriculitis in Childhood

Hiromu Yamada, Tatsuhiko Abe, Yusuke Tanabe, Noboru Sakai
Department of Neurosurgery, Gifu University School of Medicine, Gifu, Japan

Meningoventriculitis in childhood is often complicated by intraventricular septations, which may interfere with effective treatment of the disease. In order to clarify the pathogenesis of intraventricular septations and to get suggestions as to the treatment, the following experiments were performed.

Methods and Results

Experimental canine hydrocephalus was produced by intracisternal injection of 30 mg/kg of kaolin. The dogs were sacrificed 2 months after the injection and the lateral ventricular wall was observed electron microscopically. Overlying the ventricular wall proper, which had cilia and microvilli, a pseudo-membranous structure was formed, which consisted of glial cells and their mesh-like processes and was partially in continuity with the ventricular wall proper (fig. 1a). Glial proliferation was seen forming layers over the ependymal surface and passing through the ependymal layer (fig. 1b).

The finding in hydrocephalic dogs, that glial cells were growing through ependymal defect sites into the ventricular cavity, was considered to coincide with the theory of 'herniation of glial tuft', described by *Berman and Banker* [1] (cf. fig. 4b).

In the next experiments, ventriculitis was produced in rabbits by injecting 0.2 ml of *E. coli* suspension into the lateral ventricle. On the ependymal surface, pseudo-membranous structures, consisting of fibrin, blood cells and cell debris, were being formed. The pseudo-membranous structures had covered all over the ventricular surface, and tips of cilia, which originated from the ventricular wall proper, were seen to make their appearance, penetrating the pseudo-membranes (fig. 2a). The case of figure 2b was sacrificed 1 month after the first inoculation. At the site of ependymal defect, a pseudo-membranous structure, consisting of

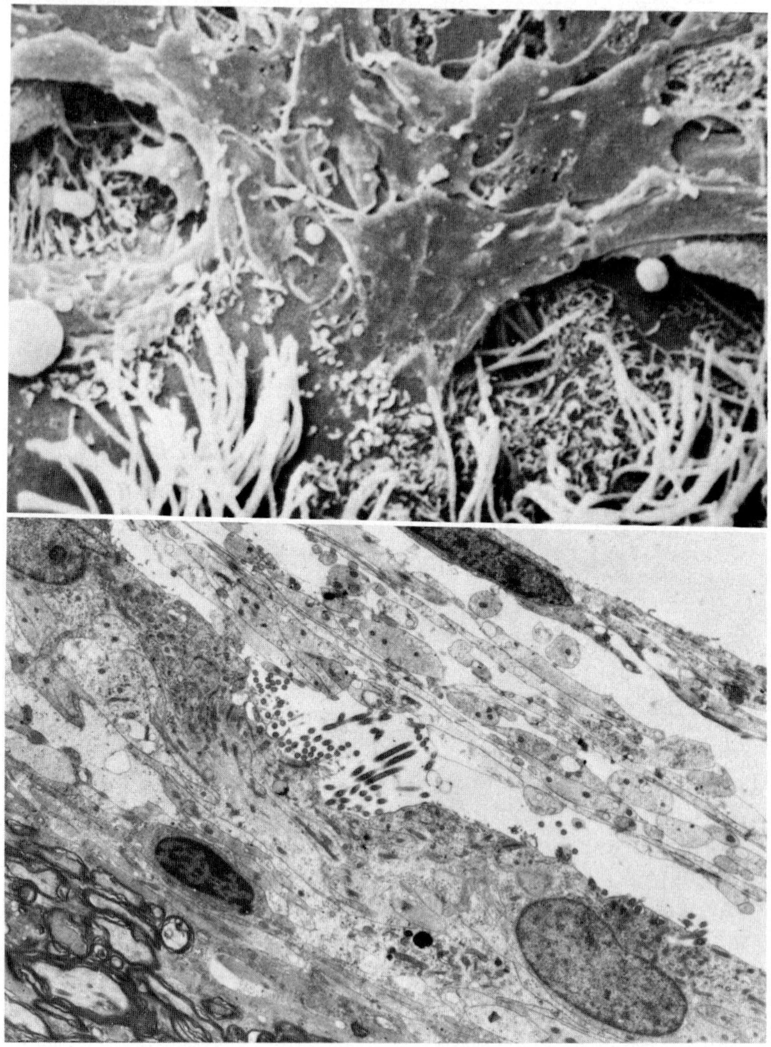

Fig. 1. In cases of experimental canine hydrocephalus. *a* A pseudo-membranous structure was formed over the ventricular wall proper (SEM). *b* Glial proliferation was seen forming layers over the ependymal surface (TEM).

fibrin and cell debris, was formed. Glial cells were seen to extend along the pseudo-membranous structure, and some of them were seen to protrude into the ventricular cavity.

The finding in ventriculitis rabbits, that glial cells were growing toward accumulation of inflammatory products, was in accordance with the theory of

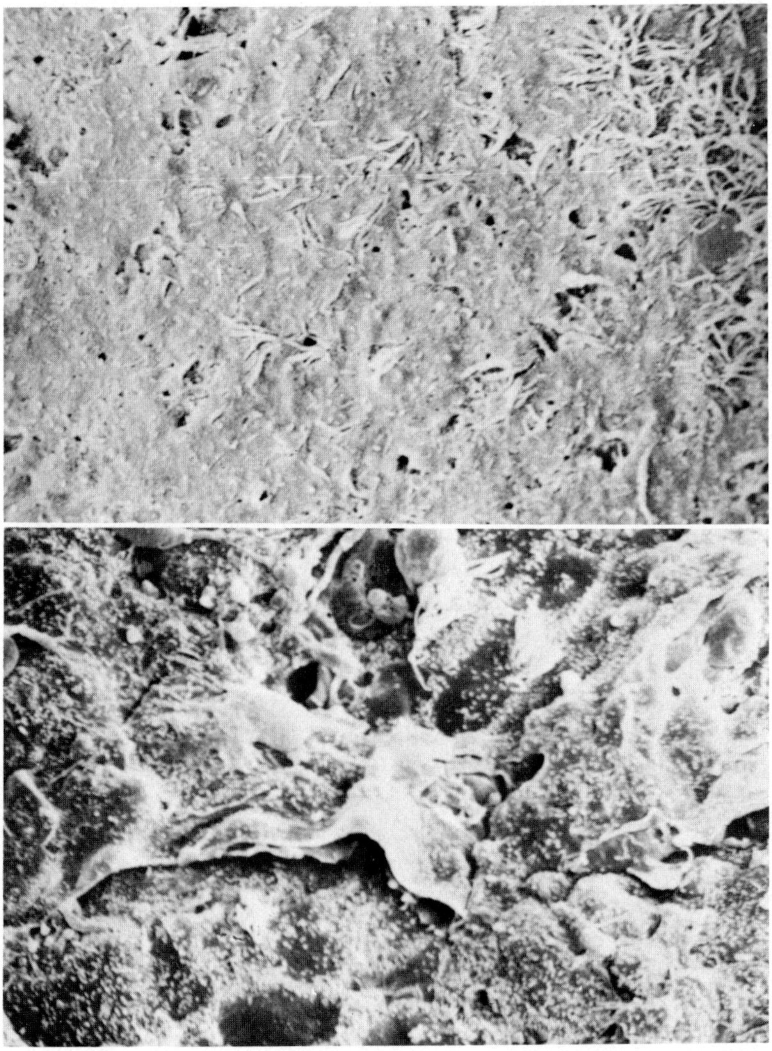

a

b

Fig. 2. In cases of experimental rabbit ventriculitis. *a* The pseudo-membranous structure had covered all over the ventricular surface, and tips of cilia were seen to make their appearance, penetrating the pseudo-membranes (SEM). *b* At the site of ependymal defect, a pseudo-membranous structure, consisting of fibrin, cell debris and glial cells, was formed (SEM).

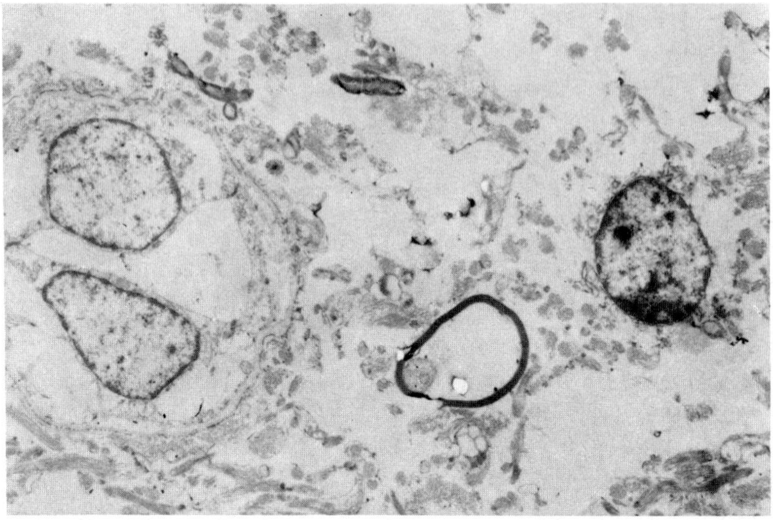

Fig. 3. TEM of intraventricular septation in a 9-year-old female case of infected hydrocephalus, revealed the existence of a myelinated fiber.

'tuft formation by organization of inflammatory products' by *Schultz and Leeds* [4] (cf. fig. 4c).

In clinical cases, most intraventricular septations are supposed to be formed by such mechanisms. They are to be prevented, not only by early eradication of infection, but also by cleansing as far as possible intraventricular inflammatory products, which possibly are the inducer of glial tufts, by means of such procedures as external ventricular drainage, intraventricular irrigation and drainage through a ventricular reservoir, or continuous intraventricular irrigation with dilute antibiotic solution.

Clinical Case

We experienced a 9-year-old female case of infected hydrocephalus, which succumbed to the infection. At autopsy, the brain showed multiple cystic formations, some apparently originating from the ventricles and others apparently porencephalic in nature. They were bordered with each other by complete or incomplete septations. The specimen, which was taken from a septation in the region of the lateral ventricle, appeared, at a glance, to be a glial tuft. Electron microscopy of the same formalin-preserved specimen revealed the existence of a myelinated fiber (fig. 3). Thus, this septation appeared at first to be an intraventricularly formed glial tuft, but it actually was found to be the brain parenchyme, which remained between the ventricle and a porencephalic cyst produced closely adjacent to the ventricle. We think this type of septation should be included in intraventricular septations in a wide sense [3] (cf. fig. 4d).

a

b

c

d

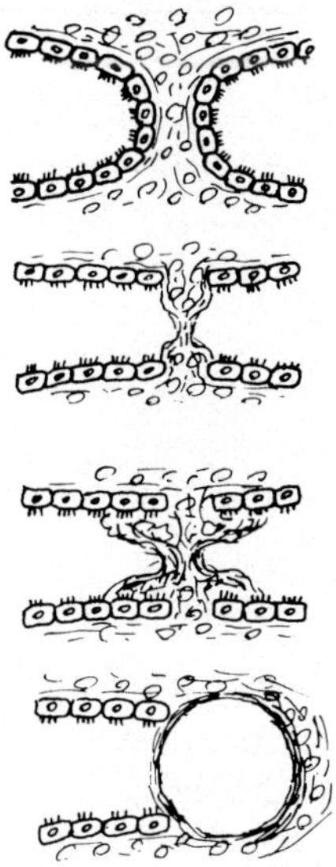

Fig. 4. Proposed pathogenetic classification of intraventicular septations. *a* Synechia consisting of astrocytes and ependyma due to proliferation of germinal cells [2]. *b* Herniation of glial tufts at the sites of ependymal defects [1]. *c* Fibroglial tufts resulting from organisation of inflammatory products [4]. *d* Brain tissues remaining between the ventricle and a porencephalic cyst close to the ventricle.

Conclusion

Including these types and the type of fibrous astrocytic synechiae, which was originally described by *Clark and Milhorat* [2] (cf. fig. 4a), we propose classification of intraventricular septations into these 4 types (fig. 4).

References

1 Berman, P.H.; Banker, B.Q.: Neonatal meningitis. A clinical and pathological study of 29 cases. Pediatrics, Springfield *38:* 6–24 (1966).

2 Clark, R.G.; Milhorat, T.H.: Experimental hydrocephalus. Light microscopic findings in acute and subacute obstructive hydrocephalus in the monkey. J. Neurosurg. *32:* 400–413 (1970).

3 Sakata, K.; Yamada, H.; Funakoshi, T.; Abe, T.: On pathogenesis of intraventricular septations (in Japanese). Nerv. Syst. Childhood *3:* 295–302 (1978).

4 Schultz, P.; Leeds, N.E.: Intraventricular septations complicating neonatal meningitis. J. Neurosurg. *38:*620–626 (1973).

H. Yamada, MD, Department of Neurosurgery, Gifu University School of Medicine, Gifu (Japan)

Other Complications

Monogr. neural Sci., vol. 8, pp. 86–87 (Karger, Basel 1982)

Lecture

K. Shulman

Albert Einstein College of Medicine, Bronx, N.Y., USA

The complications of shunting can include the appearance of subdural collections and an isolated fourth ventricle. Both of these conditions occur rarely and there is only minimal data currently available on the incidence of either condition in a large number of children with well-established shunts. With regard to the subdural collection definitions and terminology are important. The diagnosis has largely been made on CT evidence without clinical symptoms of a subdural hematoma. The exception is the older child who is shunted for the first time and develops brain collapse with dire consequences [2]. It has been postulated that overdrainage of cerebrospinal fluid in certain children causes the appearance of subdural fluid and one could ask the question whether children with certain types of hydrocephalus are more prone to develop such effusions. On theoretical grounds alone one could argue that those with large surface subarachnoid spaces would be more apt to develop the subdural collection in response to the creation of space over the surface secondary to the drainage of such large subarachnoid spaces. It does not appear that the technique of hunting nor the distal position of the shunt nor the type of valve is related in a causal fashion nor is there any shunt system which prevents this event from occurring in a small number of patients. The effusions are generally not filled with blood or red blood cell products on CT examination. Reports of the protein content of the effusion oftentimes show little difference between such protein content and that of cerebrospinal fluid. *Sato* [4] has shown passage of CSF tagged with isotope from the subarachnoid space to the subdural collection in some infants. The membranes which develop in the subdural space following shunting usually lack the proliferating character with neovasculature seen after bleeding. *McLone et al.* [3] believe that this lack probably indicates that such lesions are not progressive. *Emery* [1] has described a thickening of the arachnoid and an augmentation of the subdural tissue, acting as a space filler, after shunting. The importance from the pathophysiology point of view is whether these spaces have a pressure higher than general intracranial pressure or ventricular pressure. Attempts to measure surface subarachnoid pressure and ventricular pressure in unshunted hydrocephalics has generally yielded simultaneous pressures without a significant pressure gradient. Again there is no data on pressure differences between the subdural effusion and the pressure of the shunt which is general intracranial pressure on a child after shunt placement.

This issue of pressure gradients is also raised with regard to the isolated fourth ventricle. Here, one deals with a ventricle with higher pressure than that of the lateral ventricles containing the shunt. *Sorensen and Gaab* [5] have measured a pressure difference of 4–6 Torr between supra and infratentorial epidural pressure in a few infants with the Dandy-Walker abnormality. Such a pressure difference suggests that both the lateral ventricle and the posterior fossa cyst should be shunted. The development of an isolated fourth ventricle after shunting seems to be capable of causing similar pressure gradients across the tentorium. Once a loculated fluid collection develops in the posterior fossa, as with an isolated fourth ventricle, small volume increases in that ventricle can result in symptoms because of the limited volume buffering capacity of the small posterior fossa. Certainly the beneficial results of shunting an isolated fourth ventricle with relief and reversal of symptoms presented in this symposium provide further evidence for such pressure gradients within the head.

References

1 Emery, J.L.: Intracranial effects of long-standing decompression of the brain in children with hydrocephalus meningomyelocele. Devl Med. Child Neurol. 302–309 (1965).

2 Hovind, K.H.: Subdural hematoma as a complication in shunt-dependent hydrocephalus. Proc. Int. Soc. Ped. Neurosurgery, Marseilles (1980).

3 McLone, D.G.; Gutierrez, F.A.; Wiederhold, M.: The ultrastructure of subdural membranes of children. Proc. Int. Soc. Ped. Neurosurgery, Marseilles (1980).

4 Sato, K.; The role of cerebrospinal fluid in the development of infantile subdural effusions. Proc. Int. Soc. Ped. Neurosurgery, Marseilles (1980).

5 Sorensen, N.; Gaab, M.; Supra and infratentorial epidural pressure monitoring in Dandy-Walker syndrome. Proc. Int. Soc. Ped. Neurosurgery, Marseilles (1980).

K. Shulman, MD, Albert Einstein College of Medicine, Bronx, NY (USA)

Monogr. neural Sci., vol. 8, pp. 88–89 (Karger, Basel 1982)

Subdural Collection after Shunting Procedure in Hydrocephalic Children – with Special Reference to the Method of Shunting Procedure

Keiji Koshu, Akira Takaku, Kazuo Mizoi, Takamasa Kayama, Takashi Yoshimoti, Namio Kodama, Jiro Suzuki

Division of Neurosurgery, Institute of Brain Diseases, Tohoku University School of Medicine, Sendai, Japan

Introduction

We have experienced 110 shunting procedures in internal hydrocephalic infants in the past 15 years. Subdural collection was seen in 7 of these cases. We now analyse the cases and report some problems.

Analysis of the Cases

During the past 15 years (1965–1979), we performed 110 shunting procedures in infants. 7 of these cases showed postoperative subdural collection (6.4%). Shunting procedures were performed between 1 and 25 months after delivery. The interval between the time of shunting operation and that of diagnosis is between 4 days and 2 years. 2 cases were diagnosed by CT scan on the 4th and 7th day after shunting operation, respectively. The other 5 cases were diagnosed much later by angiography.

In the 1960s, ventriculo-atrial shunt (VAS) was performed in our clinic, but since 1971 ventriculoperitoneal shunt (VPS) has been performed. Subdural collection was seen in 5 of the 45 VAS cases, and 2 of the 65 VPS cases. The mean value of the opening pressure of slit valves was 58 mm H_2O in the subdural collection group. On the other hand, the mean value in the normal groups was 83 mm H_2O. Meningitis was seen in 3 cases before or after the shunting operations. These cases revealed the formation of membrane, and had relatively high protein content in the subdural fluid.

We treated the patients by irrigation in 3 cases, and subduroperitoneal shunt (SPS) in 2 cases. CT scans of 1 typical case who was cured by SPS are shown in figure 1. Bilateral large subdural collection disappeared on the 4th day

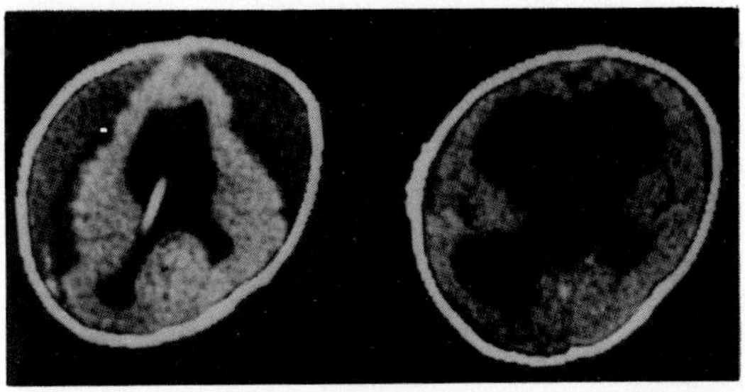

Fig. 1. CT scans taken before (left) and after SPS (right).

after SPS. 1 patient was diagnosed as having subdural collection on angiography. His symptom was, however, not as severe, therefore he was kept under careful observation. 1 year later, subdural collection was no longer found on angiography.

Another patient was treated by VAS at the age of 6 months. At the age of 6 years, abnormal calcification was detected at the left temporoparietal area. An avascular area was also seen on angiography. On operation, thickened membrane and old hematoma were found. After removal of the hematoma, SPS was set. Her mental retardation, however, did not improve after the operation.

Discussion

Our retrospective study revealed that the incidence in the VPS group was low in comparison to that in the VAS group. As for the opening pressure, valves having lower pressure were used in the subdural collection group. To prevent the formation of subdural collection, it is better to choose a VPS apparatus with a relatively high opening pressure.

Nowadays anti-syphon valves are widely used and the incidence of subdural collection decreased.

Subdural collection after shunting procedures can be detected relatively easily in the early stages by means of CT scan. In such cases SPS is generally effective if its opening pressure is lower than that of VPS. But when detected at a rather late stage, it is quite troublesome. Further efforts concerning this condition are necessary in the treatment of these patients.

K. Koshu, MD, Division of Neurosurgery, Institute of Brain Diseases,
Tohoku University School of Medicine, Sendai (Japan)

Monogr. neural Sci., vol. 8, pp. 90–91 (Karger, Basel 1982)

Subdural Collections after Shunting Procedure in Children

Etiology, Treatment and Results

J. Montaut, L. Picard, J. Roland, A. Czorny, K. Saboori
Service de Neurochirurgie 'B' (Prof. *J. Montaut*), Nancy, France

This paper is concerned with chronic subdural effusions developing in hydrocephalic children treated with ventriculoperitoneal or ventriculo-atrial shunts. The children presenting no signs of increased intracranial pressure and where the volume of the effusion is constant and the shunt patent have been excluded from this study. We also exclude from this study the subdural collections of the adults treated by ventriculo-atrial shunt for a chronic hydrocephalus with late decompensation.

The global frequency of subdural hematomas in children with non-tumoral hydrocephalus was 12 cases out of 305, that is 4% during the 10 last years. The etiology of the hydrocephalus seemed to have no influence on the occurrence of subdural hematomas.

Predisposing factors to the development of subdural hematomas are evident. The occurrence is more frequent in children over the age of 2 in our material when the fontanelles are always closed: in children under the age of 2, subdural hematomas have developed in 5 cases out of 255 (2%); in children over the age of 2, subdural hematomas have developed in 7 cases out of 50 (14%). There is an increased risk of subdural hematomas with increased skull circumference.

The ventricles were extremely large. The opening pressure of the shunt tube valve has to be considered: 5 children have a low opening pressure valve and 7 have a medium opening pressure valve. We have never seen a subdural hematoma in children with high opening pressure valves.

The diagnosis is easy because all cases have clinical signs and symptoms: in 9 cases, signs of intracranial hypertension were present (5 headaches, 5 vomiting, 3 consciousness disturbances); 1 case showed hypotonia; 1 case had a psychomotor retardation, and 1 case showed an increase of the skull circumference. These signs have developed mostly within 3 months after the shunt operation: 5 cases within 1 month; 4 cases within 1–3 months, and 3 cases within 2–4 years postoperatively. The most informative neuroradiological examination is late CT

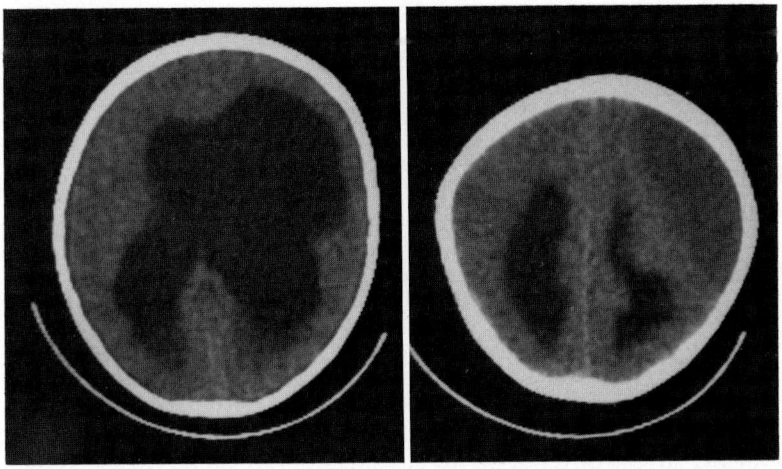

a b

Fig. 1. a Hydrocephaly prevailing at the left side before shunt. *b* After ventriculo-peritoneal shunt: left ventricular collapse and unilateral subdural effusion.

scan. The significant signs are an extensive ventricular collapse and cortical detachment which increases with time (fig. 1).

Many treatments have been tried, and we have used only two different therapeutic approaches: in some cases, surgical treatment of the hematoma and temporary suppression of the shunt; this was performed in 10 out of 12 cases. It is a highly efficient treatment for the hematoma. The risk is a rapid development of intracranial hypertension due to the ventricular dilatation. In these cases we were obliged to apply a new shunt within 2–6 days. In 2 cases, we had intracranial hypertension within 24 h and death. In some other cases, surgical treatment of the hematoma with preservation of the shunt was performed (2 cases). This treatment produced a recurrence of the hematoma and implies a modification of the shunt into a high opening pressure valve.

Results of treatment in 12 cases: successful, 7; neurologic sequelae, 2; death, 3 (acute intracranial hypertension, 2; infection, 1).

Prof. J. Montaut, Service de Neurochirurgie 'B', Hôpital Saint-Julien,
C.O. No 34, F–54037 Nancy Cédex (France)

Monogr. neural Sci., vol. 8, pp. 92–95 (Karger, Basel 1982)

Post-Shunt Porencephaly – as a Complication of Shunt in Hydrocephalus

K. Fujita, H. Hirayama, T. Kusunoki, N. Tamaki, S. Matsumoto

Department of Neurological Surgery, Kobe University, School of Medicine, Kobe, Japan

With the advent of CT scan, the abnormalities in the ventricular system and cerebral parenchyma appear to be better outlined and more easily by CT scan than by other neuroradiological procedures. In the diagnosis of porencephaly, CT scan has been of particular value, since other neuroradiological procedures have not been helpful. The aim of this report is to present the clinical manifestations and CT findings in 11 cases of post-shunt porencephaly and to comment the mechanism on the occurrence of post-shunt porencephaly.

Case Materials

We reviewed pre- and post-shunt CT scans of 156 hydrocephalic patients obtained on the EMI head scanner. Post-shunt porencephaly was diagnosed by comparison of CT findings in hydrocephalic patients obtained before and after shunt, excluding the cases of congenital porencephaly associated with hydrocephalus. 11 cases of post-shunt porencephaly were presented with a description of the clinical data, CT scan and follow-up results in these patients.

Results

Clinical findings in the post-shunt porencephalic cases are summarized in table I. The shunt was revised once due to malfunction with the exception of 1 case, but in most cases, the frequency of shunt revision was from 2 to 5 times. A ventricular catheter was introduced from the right or left occipital area, aiming at the trigone of the lateral ventricles, with the exception of 2 cases in whom the catheter was introduced from the frontal area. Post-shunt porencephaly was diagnosed by comparison of the CT scan before and after shunt, excluding the congenital porencephaly, and was frequently found 1 or 2 years after the shunt

Table I. Clinical summary of 11 cases of post-shunt porencephaly

Case	Age, years	Sex	Diagnosis	Neurological findings	Location of cyst	Convulsion	Developmental retardation
1	3	F	MMC + hydrocephalus	paraparesis and sphincter disturbance	right occipito-temporal area	hemiconvulsion	(–)
2	7	F	MMC + hydrocephalus	paraparesis and sphincter disturbance	left occipital area	hemiconfulsion	(–)
3	10	M	congenical hydro-cephalus	mental retardation left hemiparesis	right occipital area	generalized seizure	slight mental retardation
4	2	F	MMC + hydrocephalus	paraparesis and spincter disturbance	left parietal area	(–)	(–)
5	1	F	post-hemorrhagic hydrocephalus	mental retardation hemiconvulsion	right temporo-parietal area	hemiconvulsion	slight mental retardation
6	6	F	post-meningitic hydrocephalus	developmental retardation quadriparesis	right frontal area	generalized seizure	marked developmental retardation
7	10	M	congenital hydro-cephalus	left hemiparesis	right occipital area	generalized seizure	moderate develop-mental retardation
8	8	M	congenital hydro-cephalus	left hemiparesis visual disturbance	right frontal area	(–)	slight developmental retardation
9	1.5	F	hydrocephalus + subdural effusion	IICP	left frontal area	(–)	(–)
10	3	F	congenital hydro-cephalus	marked developmental retardation	right occipital area	generalized seizure	marked developmental retardation
11	6	F	MMC + hydrocephalus	paraparesis and sphincter disturbance	right occipital area	(–)	(–)

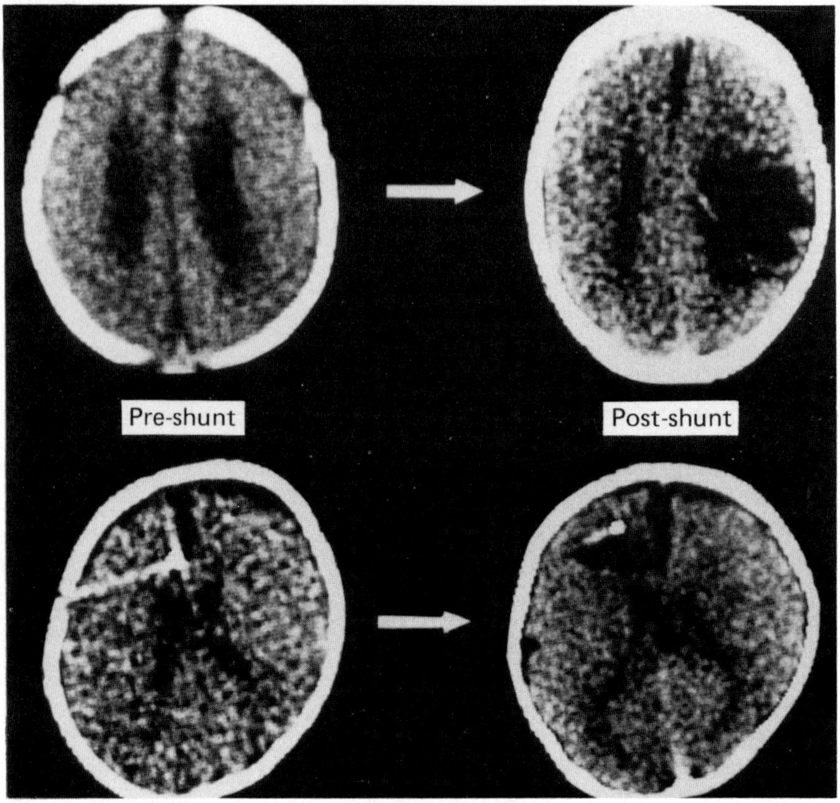

Fig. 1. Pre-shunt and post-shunt porencephaly.

in hydrocephalic cases in whom the shunt was placed during the age of 1 year, as shown in figure 1. When porencephaly was divided into 2 groups according to its size, large porencephaly was more frequently found.

As to the clinical manifestations, the patients have symptoms and signs of local or generalized cerebral disease. Convulsions, delayed development and focal motor deficits are the most common clinical findings. Visual signs were difficult to evaluate but 3 patients seem to have contralateral hemianopia. As to the type of seizure, all patients showed generalized or focal seizure. An electroencephalogram is a valuable aid in the diagnosis of porencephaly. All cases had this study performed with 9 being abnormal. There was a high degree of correlation between the site of local EEG changes, the location and the size of the cysts. 6 patients were mentally and pysically retarded with marked developmental retardation in 2 patients. But there seems to be no correlation between the degree of developmental retardation and the presence of post-shunt porencephaly or the size of the porencephaly.

Discussion

Shunt procedures have been routinely performed for the treatment of hydrocephalus in many institutes and many reports dealing with shunt complications, such as shunt infection, subdural hematoma or shunt malfunction, are available in the literature. However, reports of post-shunt porencephaly as a complication of shunt are quite few. With the advent of the CT scan, porencephaly can readily be recognized. Especially the areas of closed porencephaly which would be missed by other modalities are readily diagnosed by the CT scan. Most porencephaly is congenital but it might frequently be acquired in infants. Post-shunt porencephaly is also an acquired type of porencephaly, mainly due to a combination of trauma and inflammation, in addition to the mechanical factor of the cerebrospinal fluid. Acquired porencephaly is usually the result of the cerebral tissue destruction from various causes, such as trauma, vascular insufficiency or infection. Post-shunt porencephaly, although sometimes silent, may progress in size and often causes a variety of clinical symptoms, such as developmental retardation, increased intracranial pressure signs, seizure and motor deficit, and a large cyst in post-shunt porencephaly situated near the motor cortex often causes seizure and motor deficit. These facts justify a more vigorous attempt to prevent these complications at early diagnosis. From our clinical data of 11 cases, the etiologic factors in the formation of post-shunt porencephaly might be considered as follows: (1) surgical trauma due to a frequent puncture of the ventricle may be initiating factors; (2) the ventricular catheter may cause mechanical irritation due to cerebral pulsation and also a foreign body reaction to the brain substance, and (3) most of post-shunt porencephalic cases are shunt-dependent hydrocephalus. Increased intraventricular pressure due to shunt malfunction may be a promoting factor.

K. Fujita, MD, Department of Neurological, Surgery, Kobe University, School of Medicine, Kobe (Japan)

Monogr. neural Sci., vol. 8, pp. 96–98 (Karger, Basel 1982)

The Isolated Fourth Ventricle: A Complication of Shunting of the Lateral Ventricles in Children

Giuseppe Scotti[a], *Charles R. Fitz*[b], *Derek C. Harwood-Nash*[b], *Mark A. Musgrave*[b]

[a]Università di Milano, Ospedale Policlinico, Clinica Neurologica, Milano, Italy; [b]Department of Radiology, The Hospital for Sick Children, Toronto, Ont. Canada Toronto, Ont. Canada

Among the complications of lateral ventricular shunting the isolated fourth ventricle is a rare event. It may occur when, due to mechanical or inflammatory causes, both the aqueduct of Sylvius and the foramina of Luschka and Magendie become occluded, thus isolating the fourth ventricle from the remaining ventricular system and from the CSF circulation of the subarachnoid space. Continued CSF production by the trapped choroid plexus results in a progressive cystic dilatation of the fourth ventricle which is sometimes associated with clinical signs of an expanding lesion in the posterior fossa. Shunting of the isolated fourth ventricle may result in complete disappearance of the symptoms.

Raimondi et al. [1] first reported 4 cases among 8 with Dandy-Walker syndrome in whom shunting of the lateral ventricles had resulted in occlusion of a previously patent aqueduct with the appearance of new signs of posterior fossa mass lesion, thus requiring a separate shunt in the 'encysted Dandy-Walker cyst'. These patients however already had a congenital malformation of the fourth ventricle. The very first report of an isolated fourth ventricle must thus be considered that of *DeFeo et al.* [2] in 1975. Since then other papers have been published on the subject [3, 4]; we have recently reported our experience with 16 children with this condition diagnosed by CT at the Hospital for Sick Children of Toronto [5].

All the children had been previously shunted for different types of hydrocephalus at different ages. All patients had had multiple shunt revisions and a high incidence of shunt infections.

The diagnosis of isolated fourth ventricle was made on the basis of CT findings in all patients. A large rounded or pear-shaped midline cystic structure was present in the posterior fossa (fig. 1a). The lateral and third ventricles were small or only moderately enlarged (fig. 1b).

In only 7 of the 16 patients immediate pre-CT posterior fossa signs charac-

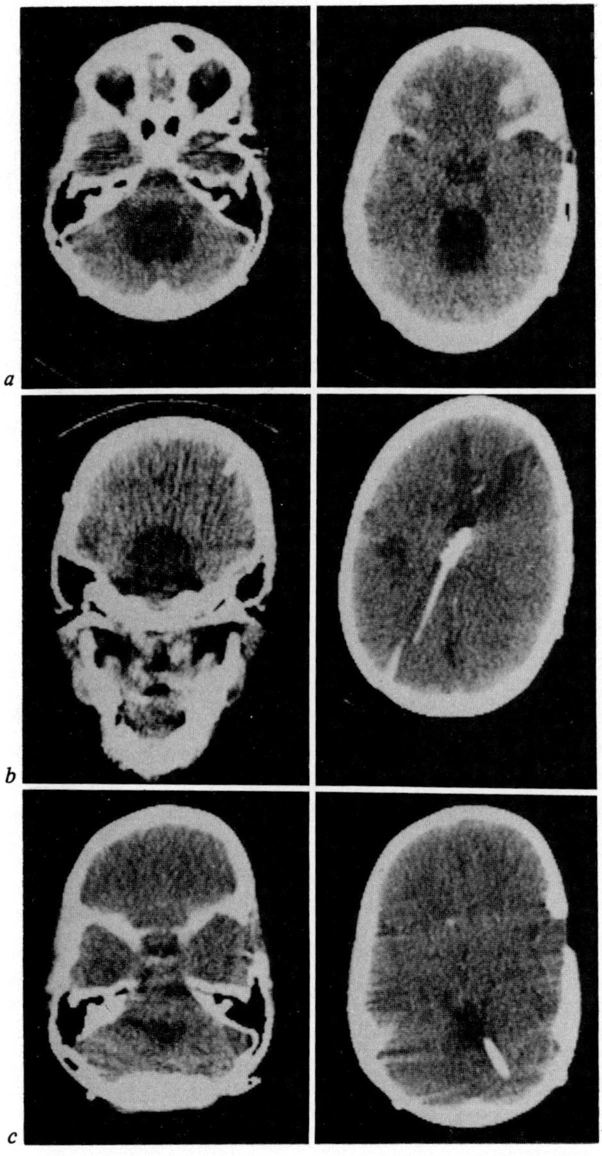

Fig. 1. a–c A typical case of an isolated fourth ventricle in a 6-year-old child, shunted for extraventricular obstructive hydrocephalus following intraventricular haemorrhage at birth. Multiple shunts and shunt revisions. The fourth ventricle is very large and well demonstrated both in axial (*a*) and coronal (*b*) views. The shunted lateral ventricles are small (*b*). After shunting (*c*) the fourth ventricle has returned to normal size.

terized by ataxia, diplopia and increasing lethargy were evident and, in one of them, only in retrospect.

In 14 patients a shunt was inserted directly into the isolated fourth (fig. 1c), producing good results in 6, with the posterior fossa signs clearing completely or in part.

On the basis of our experience we may state that the clinical presentation of this entity is rarely in the form of the full-blown posterior fossa syndrome characterized by a recent appearance of ataxia, diplopia and increasing drowsiness without raised intracranial pressure. Signs of posterior fossa involvement may be present for years without being progressive; the isolated fourth may even be asymptomatic and discovered at CT as an incidental finding. In some cases pre-existing neurological signs such as spasticity, hemi- or quadriparesis may be accentuated without the appearance of posterior fossa signs.

Shunting of the fourth ventricle is effective in rapidly reversing the posterior fossa signs when they are present and progressive. In other cases there may be some relief of pre-existing neurological signs or no change at all, despite a demonstrable decrease in the size of the shunted fourth ventricle. The fourth ventricular shunt is subject to the same problems as any shunt elsewhere in the ventricular system. It may malfunction causing reenlargement of the fourth ventricle. The lateral ventricular shunt may malfunction while the shunt in the fourth ventricle is working well.

Since this is, in some cases at least, a potentially curable entity, a CT scan should be performed on all patients with shunted hydrocephalus who develop new posterior fossa signs or worsening of pre-existing neurological deficits. The CT diagnosis of isolated fourth ventricle is accurate and can be made without recourse to metrizamide ventriculography. When the diagnosis is made, the lateral ventricles are usually normal in size or only moderately dilated.

The term isolated fourth ventricle should be reserved for the type of patients we have described. When the fourth ventricle is larger than usual in association with hydrocephalus but returns to normal after shunting of the lateral ventricles, the term 'disproportionately large, communicating fourth ventricle' should be used.

References

1 Raimondi, A.J.; Samuelson, G.; Yarzgaray, L., Norton, T.: Atresia of the foramina of Luschka and Magendie: The Dandy-Walker cyst. J. Neurosurg. *31:* 202–216 (1969).

2 DeFeo, D.; Foltz, E.L.; Hamilton, A.E.: Double compartment hydrocephalus in a patient with cysticercosis meningitis. Surg. Neurol, *4:* 247–251 (1975).

3 Zimmerman, R.A.; Bilaniuk, L.T.; Galli, E.: Computed tomography of the trapped fourth ventricle. Am. J. Roentg. *130:* 503–506 (1978).

4 Hawkins, J.C.; Hoffman, H.J.; Humphreys, R.P.: Isolated fourth ventricle as a complication of ventricular shunting. J. Neurosurg. *49:* 910–913 (1978).

5 Scotti, G.; Musgrave, M.A.; Fitz, C.R.; Harwood-Nash, D.C.: The isolated fourth ventricle in children: a CT and clinical review of sixteen cases. AJNR *1:* 419–424 (1980).

Dr. G. Scotti, Università di Milano, Ospedale Policlinico, Clinica Neurologica, Via F. Sforza 35, I–20122 Milano (Italy)

Monogr. neural Sci., vol. 8, pp. 99–101 (Karger, Basel 1982)

Craniostenosis Secondary to Ventricular Shunt

Akira Yokota, Yasuhiko Matsukado

Department of Neurosurgery, Kumamoto University Medical School, Kumamoto, Japan

While the early complications due to reduction of the intracranial pressure following shunting procedures for infantile hydrocephalus are well documented, long-term effects of the procedure have recently been recognized to offer some distortions on the developing brain and skull. Craniostenosis secondary to the shunt operation is considered one of such chronic complications. The authors have observed 3 cases of secondary craniostenosis out of 75 shunted infants within the last 10 years follow-up and 2 representative cases among them are shown in this paper.

Case 1. The 2-year-3month-old girl was delivered prematurely at 9 months with a birth weight of 1,950 g and a head circumference of 31.5 cm. Hydrocephalus appeared around the age of 30 days when the head circumference was measured 41.5 cm. Skull films showed marked separation of all cranial sutures and an air study demonstrated symmetrical hydrocephalus in an advanced stage due to aqueductal stenosis. Thickness of the brain mantle in the frontal region was measured 0.5 cm. Ventriculo-atrial shunt was performed with a Pudenz medium-pressure valve at the age of 45 days. The patient was readmitted at the age of 2 years and 3 months because of visual difficulty and papilledema. Examination disclosed severe developmental retardation and oxycephalic deformity with a head circumference of 44.0 cm. The shunt was found not to function. On the skull film marked digital markings and closure of all cranial sutures were demonstrated. Linear craniectomy was carried out for secondary craniosynostosis, and it was followed by shunt revision because of subsequent bulging of the head. After a series of interventions the patient lived an uneventful life, still marked in developmental retardation, and the death was reported 1 year later.

Case 2. The 9-year-old boy. Hydrocephalus appeared spontaneously around the age of 4 months, when the radiological examinations disclosed symmetrical hydrocephalus of advanced stage with a cortical cerebral mantle of 1 cm thickness. Ventriculo-atrial shunt and its revisions with a Pudenz medium-pressure valve were performed during the first 1.5 years. For the following 8 years the patient showed sufficient physical development and retained an IQ score above 100, though the head circumference remained below –2 SD (49 cm at the age of 9). The patient was brachycephalic and prominent coronal synostosis was demonstrated on the skull film. Shunt dysfunction had been pointed out since the age of 4 without any clinical symptoms and his hydrocephalus had been considered to be arrested. At the age of 9 the patient complained of severe headache particularly early in the morning. Findings on CT scans were much the same as before for the last 2 years, which showed mild symmetrical dilatation of the cerebral ventricles. Finally retinal hemorrhage was noticed and continuous recording of the intraventricular pressure demonstrated transcient elevations of the intracranial pressure corresponding to Lundgerg's B-wave early in the morning. Lineal craniectomy was performed and the patient's symptoms of intracranial hypertension improved well. The head circumference recovered within normal range in the following period.

Discussion

Considerable cases of secondary premature synostosis following shunting procedures have been reported [1–6] since this rare condition was pointed out by *Strenger* [7] in his article concerning shunt complications.

A review of 17 reported cases of secondary craniostenosis reveals the common clinical pictures as follows: (1) Hydrocephalus is extremely advanced. (2) Most of the patients are shunted within 3 months of age and secondary craniostenosis appears within 2.5 years after the initial shunting procedure. (3) Developmental retardation is the accompanying symptom of these hydrocephalic infants and their prognosis is proved to be poor even after the cranioplasty. (4) Shunt method is exclusively ventriculo-atrial/jugular. These facts indicate two main factors contributing to produce premature craniosynostosis after the shunting procedure. The principal problem is the developmental potentiality of the shunted brain. A close correlation between the intellecutal development and the cranial modifications after the shunting procedure has been well discussed [8, 9]. Shunted children with permissible intelligence retain skulls of normal shape and of size in physiological range; however, notable radiological abnormalities of the skull such as premature synostosis are found in retarded children [9]. Impaired growth of the brain or failed restoration of the cerebral mantle after shunt operation settles the intracranial condition in low pressure, which promotes thickening and sclerosis of the cranial bones and sutures. Thus, the cranial modifications represented by premature synostosis largely depend on the development of the shunted brain.

The second point is the pressure-reducing effect of the shunting procedure. In the case of advanced hydrocephalus, sudden and persistent reduction of the intracranial pressure easily brings on overlapping of the cranial sutures, which also promotes premature synostosis. *Anderson* [1] pointed out that this complication followed much frequently with placement of the low-pressure valve, but it cannot always be avoided by the use of medium pressure valve from our experience. It is of interest that secondary craniosynostosis has not been known so far in the patients treated with the ventriculoperitoneal shunt. This may be explained by the fact that the pressure-reducing effect of the ventriculo-atrial shunt is greater than that of the ventriculoperitoneal shunt particularly in the younger infant.

However, all the shunted children with premature synostosis do not necessarily present practical problems as craniostenosis, because most of them are regarded as secondary microcephaly. Only a few of the craniosynostotic patients show clinical manifestations when the shunt dysfunctions in a shunt-dependent state or when the shunted brain regains its development.

Case 1 well represents the clinical course of craniostenosis secondary to shunt operation discussed above, of which the ultimate prognosis cannot be much expected because it reflects a poor development of the shunted brain. If one evaluates it as secondary microcephaly, an indication for cranioplasty should be doubtful regardless of radiological evidence of craniosynostosis. On the contrary, a definite indication for cranioplasty should be applied for another type of secondary craniostenosis, such as case 2, of which hydrocephalus had once been assumed to be arrested for a long time with a good developmental score and with permissible recovery of the brain mantle as revealed on CT scan. This type of shunted children seems to be encountered much more frequently in the long-term follow-up, but has never been reported so far.

References

1 Anderson, H.: Craniosynostosis as a complication after operation for hydrocephalus. Acta paediat. scand. *55:* 192–196 (1966).

2 Chiba, T.; Shimizu, K.: Craniostenosis secondary to ventriculo-atrial shunt for infantile hydrocephalus. Geka-Chiryo *10:* 225–229 (1968).

3 Kloss, J.L.: Craniosynostosis secondary to ventriculo-atrial shunt. Am. J. Dis. Child. *116:* 315–317 (1968).

4 Lagrange, E.; Schäfer, H.: Verlaufsbeobachtungen bei Hydrozephalus nach Ventrikulo-Aurikulostomis. Dt. med. Wschr. *91:* 1918–1926 (1966).

5 Nicole, R.: Crâniosynostose secondaire et autres complications du drainage de l'hydrocéphalie. Annls Chir. infant. *10:* 41–46 (1969).

6 Roberts, J.R.; Rickham, P.P.: Craniosynostosis following Holter valve operation. Devl. med. Child Neurol. *12:* suppl. 22, pp. 145–149 (1970).

7 Strenger, L.: Complications of ventriculovenous shunts. J. Neurosurg. *20:* 219–224 (1963).

8 Villani, R.; Giani, S.M.; Giovenelli, M.; et al: Skull changes and intellectual status in hydrocephalic children following CSF shunting. Devl. med. Child Neurol. *18:* suppl. 37, pp. 78–81 (1976).

9 Yokota, A.; Matsukado, Y.; Secondary craniosynostosis following shunt operation. Long-term effects of shunting on the developing skull. Nerv. Syst. Child. *1:* 145–152 (1976).

A. Yokota, MD, Department of Neurosurgery, Kumamoto University, Medical School, Kumamoto 860 (Japan)

Monogr. neural Sci., vol. 8, pp. 102–104 (Karger, Basel 1982)

Acquired Craniostenosis following Ventriculoperitoneal Shunt for Hydrocephalus

Adelola Adeloye

Neurosurgery Unit, Department of Surgery, University College Hospital, Ibadan, Nigeria

Introduction

It is well known that after successful establishment of cerebrospinal fluid (CSF) shunting in hydrocephalus, changes occur in the vault [3, 4, 7, 8, 10] as well as the base [5, 6] of the skull. The vault changes described include: thickening of the inner table; absence of digital impression; thickening of the sutures and cranial asymmetry due to hypoplasia on the side of the shunt system. Reduction in sellar dimension, raised petrous ridges and planum sphenoidale are some of the modifications noted in the cranial floor.

One of the striking skull changes after CSF shunting is the development of craniostenosis, 3 cases of which were described by *Anderson* [2]. The purpose of this paper is to report 2 cases of this unusual complication which were encountered on the Neurosurgery Unit of the University College Hospital (UCH), Ibadan, Nigeria.

Case Reports

Case 1. S.Y., a Nigerian female child, was 2 months old when she first presented with hydrocephalus at our clinic in 1968. She was the product of a normal pregnancy and labour, and the first child of her young parents. On examination on July 8, 1968 she had a head circumference of 55 cm and was unable to hold up her head. There were no other abnormalities. Air ventriculography later showed large ventricles and a thin pallium of less than 1 cm thickness.

On August 3, 1968, she underwent a ventriculoperitoneal shunt operation, with Till-Dahl-Wade valve. The shunt functioned well. The immediate postoperative period was uneventful so that the child was discharged home 2 weeks after surgery.

While in her hospital bed, she preferred to lie on the back of her head most of the time. She had continued in this habit after leaving hospital. At the first follow-up clinic 6 weeks after discharge from hospital, slight overriding of the parietal bones over the frontal was noted. Her parents thereafter took her to Lagos, 150 km from Ibadan. When she was next seen at UCH, Ibadan, in July 1970, the craniostenotic head configuration had become established. At the same time, she had roving nystagmus of the blind, and retinoscopy showed that she had bilateral atrophic discs. The circumferences of the head and chest were 50 and 52 cm, respectively. There was moderate degree of limb spasticity.

It was suggested by her doctors in Lagos that we should remove 'the powerful Till-Dahl-Wade valve' to correct her anomalous craniology. Air studies contemplated were not carried out as the child once more disappeared from our clinic. We have not seen her since then.

Case 2. S.B., also a Nigerian female child, was 3 months old when she was first seen in our clinic on account or rapidly progressive hydrocephalus. She was apparently normal at birth, the first child of her parents and the product of an uneventful pregnancy and normal labour. She looked normal until the age of 2 months when her head started to get big. On examination on August 19, 1974, she had pronounced hydrocephalus with tense bulging anterior fontanelle and a head circumference of 57 cm. Air ventriculography later showed markedly dilated ventricles with very thin mantle.

On September 4, 1974, a ventriculoperitoneal shunt was established, using Till-Dahl-Wade valve. Within 48 h of operation, the anterior fontanelle softened, became flat and pulsatile and later obviously depressed. On the 3rd postoperative day, overlapping of the cranial bones was noted, the left parietal overriding the right, and the right frontal over the left. A week later, the head circumference measured 49 cm. She was discharged home on September 23, 1974.

She was brought to our clinic for follow-up in April 1975. The scaphocephalic head configuration was then established with the left parietal overriding the right, and the right frontal overriding the left. The craniofacial disproportion, now in favour of the face, as in craniostenosis, was present.

Discussion

The incidence of acquired craniostenosis following ventriculoperitoneal shunt is not known for sure. It would, however, appear to be a rarity, as the 2 cases reported here were the only examples encountered in our series of 154 ventriculoperitoneal shunts performed on hydrocephalic Nigerian children in our unit between 1962 and 1974 [1]. Both patients who developed postoperative craniostenosis were females, the significance of the sex bias being unknown.

Advanced rapidly progressing hydrocephalus and the use of a low-pressure valve for CSF shunting would appear to predispose to the development of acquired craniostenosis. A cortical thickness of about 1 cm noted in our cases was also reported by *Anderson* [2]. All his 3 cases had Holter valves, 2 of them of low pressure. The Till-Dahl-Wade valve used in our cases has an even lower opening pressure of 2–5 mm H_2O [9].

When it occurs, acquired craniostenosis is usually noticeable within some days or a few weeks of surgery, and it becomes established in a matter of months. Such a course of events is exemplified by our 2 cases and case 1 of *Anderson* [2]. What type of craniostenosis is acquired may be resolved by mechanical factors, depending on the position of the head in bed and the deformation suffered in the immediate postoperative period.

Blindness in acquired craniostenosis is not easy to explain. After adequate decompression of the lateral ventricles, *Emery* [4] noted that the cerebellum rises to form a tumour in the centre of the skull. As a result there is gross distortion of the occipital poles accompanied by degeneration of the occipital cortex which overlies the cerebellar mass. These pathological changes could cause cortical blindness if the visual centre in the occipital lobes is affected. In our case 1, with atrophic discs, the blindness probably resulted from damage to the optic nerves. Changes in the base of the skull might have stretched and damaged the optic nerves or interfered with their blood supply.

The surgical treatment of synostosis acquired from overdrainage of the ventricles is not favoured as it is more troublesome and complicated than in the ordinary cases [2]. Its incidence may be reduced either by the early treatment of hydrocephalus when low-pressure valves are less likely to cause significant overdrainage problems or by avoiding the use of low-pressure valves in shunting advanced, rapidly progressing hydrocephalus.

References

1 Adeloye, A.; Olumide, A.A.: Abdominal complications of ventriculoperitoneal shunts in Nigerians. Int. Surg. *62:* 525–527 (1977).

2 Anderson, H.: Craniostenosis as a complication after operation for hydrocephalus Acta paediat. scand. *55:* 192–196 (1966).

3 Anderson, R.; Kieffer, S.A.; Wolfson, J.J.; Long, D.; Peterson, H.: Thickening of the skull in surgically treated hydrocephalus. Am. J. Roent. *110:* 96 (1970).

4 Emery, J.L.: Intracranial effects of long standing decompression of the brain in children with hydrocephalus and myelomeningocele. Devl Med. Child Neur. *7:* 320–309 (1965).

5 Griscom, N.T.; Oh, K.S.: The contracting skull: inward growth of the inner table as a physiologic response to the diminution of intracranial content in children. Am. J. Roentg. *110:* 106 (1970).

6 Kaufman, B.; Sandstrom, P.H.; Young, H.F.: Alteration in size and configuration of the sella turcica as the result of prolonged cerebrospinal fluid shunting. Radiology *97:* 537 (1970).

7 Kaufman, B.; Weiss, M.H., Young H.F.; Nulsen, F.E.: Effects of prolonged cerebrospinal fluid shunting on the skull and brain. J. Neurosurg. *38:* 288 (1973).

8 Moseley, J.E.; Rabinowitz, J.G.; Dziadw, R.: Hyperostosis cranii ex vacuo. Radiology *87:* 1105 (1966).

9 Till, K.: A valve for treatment of hydrocephalus. Lancet *i:* 202 (1964).

10 Villani, R.; Giani, S.M., Giovanelli, M.; Tomei, G.; Zavanone, M.L.; Motti, E.D.F.: Skull changes and intellectual status in hydrocephalus children following CSF shunting. Devl Med. Child Neur. *37:* suppl., pp. 78–81 (1976).

Prof. A. Adeloye, Neurosurgery Unit, Department of Surgery,
University College Hospital, Ibadan (Nigeria)

Monogr. neural Sci., vol. 8, pp. 105–107 (Karger, Basel 1982)

Diagnosis and Management of Arrested Hydrocephalus

Fred Epstein
New York University Medical Center, New York, N.Y., USA

Although the general dictum of 'once a shunt – always a shunt' is generally in harmony with reality, there are a few children who do not seem to require a shunt revision following primary placement. In these few cases, a neurosurgeon is faced with several issues.

The first relates to the status of the shunt, i.e. functional or nonfunctional. The second relates to the status of the hydrocephalus, i.e. active or arrested. The third issue arises if one assumes that the hydrocephalus is arrested, and this is whether or not the shunt should be removed. It is the purpose of this representation to address all of these issues.

It seems clear, on the basis of information derived from CAT scans in children with functional and nonfunctional shunts, that the common denominator to arrested hydrocephalus is at least a moderately enlarged ventricular system. Therefore, if the scan demonstrates small ventricles, one may be quite certain that the shunt is functional and that the hydrocephalus is not arrested (fig. 1). Compensated hydrocephalus evolves during the neonatal or infant stage of development, and one may be quite certain that if increased intracranial pressure makes a shunt revision necessary after the first 6 months of life, this child will be permanently shunt-dependent. Plain skull X-rays may document shunt dependency by disclosing a thickened calvarium as well as base of the skull (fig. 2).

Children who have had only one shunt, and have a moderately enlarged ventricular system, may or may not have arrested hydrocephalus. In other words, although small ventricles are synonymous with shunt dependency large ventricles are by no means equivalent to arrested hydrocephalus. It is well-known that even with a functioning shunt, an enlarged ventricular system does not always return towards normal volume. Therefore, in the latter situation, one may only state that this child may or may not be independent of the shunt. A definitive opinion in this regard is not possible without utilizing invasive diagnostic studies. Probably the most revealing one is the shunt scan which, if it demonstrates that there

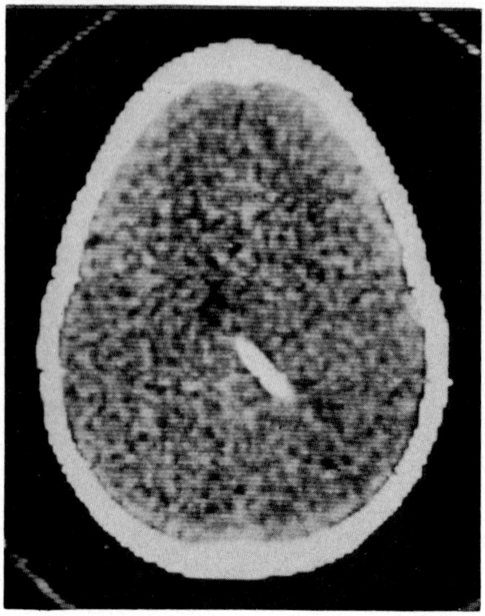

Fig. 1.

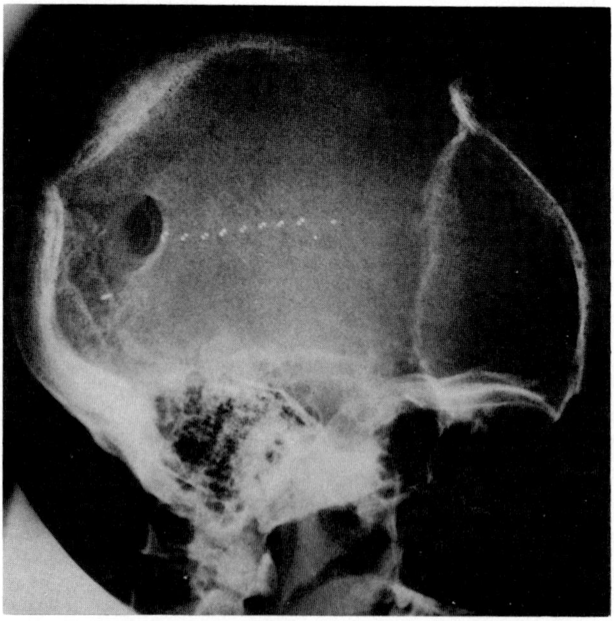

Fig. 2.

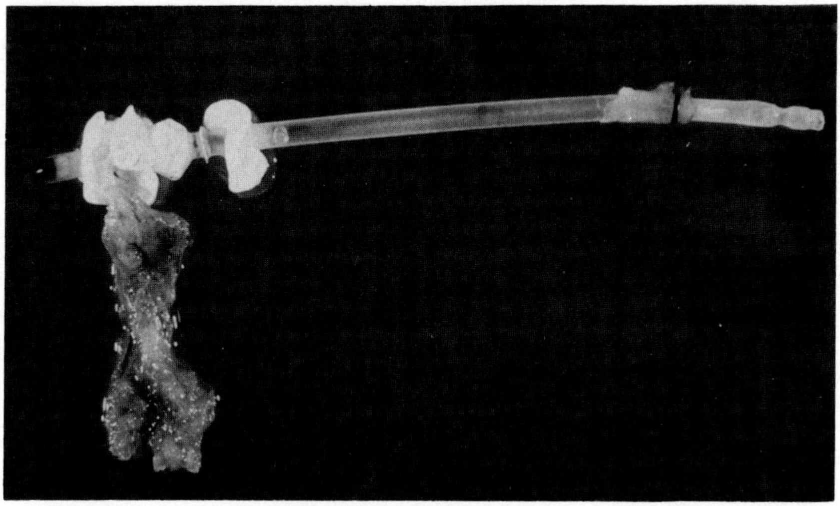

Fig. 3.

is no passage of fluid through the system in an asymptomatic child, would suggest a diagnosis of arrested hydrocephalus. It has not been our position, however, to take even small risks of infection in these children, and we recommend a course of watchful waiting. Relating to this same point, we do not advise elective lengthening of the first shunt if the child has not had one episode of obvious shunt malfunction which required revision.

It has become clear that children who have arrested hydrocephalus must be carefully monitored during the developing years. Although regular CAT scanning may document progressive ventriculomegaly it is by no means satisfactory as the only technique. This is because children may have progressive intellectual deterioration in the absence of clear-cut progressive ventriculomegaly. For this reason, it is essential that serial psychometric testing be undertaken at 12-month intervals during the first 10 years of life. Assuming that these document normal development, one may continue to pursue a course of watchful waiting in terms of following arrested hydrocephalus. If there is intellectual deterioration, the shunt must be revised.

Finally, it is the position of this author that there is no situation in which a shunt should be electively removed unless there has been a supervening spinal fluid infection. The ventricular catheter not uncommonly becomes enmeshed in the choroid plexus and a child with arrested hydrocephalus may reactivate the disease if there is even a small amount of hemorrhage within the ventricular system (fig. 3). For this reason, there is no rationale to taking a surgical risk to remove a mechanism that is causing no harm.

F. Epstein, MD, New York University Medical Center, 550 First Avenue,
New York, NY 10016 (USA)

Monogr. neural Sci., vol. 8, pp. 108–111 (Karger, Basel 1982)

Slit Ventricle – A Reluctant Goal of Ventriculoperitoneal Shunt

A. Hirayama
Kobe University School of Medicine, Kobe, Japan

Since 1968, we have been concentrating on ventriculoperitoneal shunts with a few exceptions. At first, we, our patients and their families had been enjoying the excellent and simplified control of intracranial pressure. But thereafter, we began to suffer from the problems of shunt dependency as well as other complications like infection, obstruction, etc. Recently, we have found the consequence of shunt dependency as slit ventricle clearer than in the period before CAT scan.

In this study (table I), there were 106 patients who fulfilled the following criteria: (1) ventriculoperitoneal shunts were implanted in those aged under 12 months; (2) the follow-up period at a frequency of every 3 months was not less than 12 months; (3) each patient had more than 2 CAT scans after operation which were reviewed retrospectively. In regard to the types of hydrocephalus, the criteria for congenital hydrocephalus is diagnosed within the child's first 3 months with no evidence of associated dysraphism and infections.

Death was reported in 5 cases and, although no postmortem examination was allowed, these deaths might have been related to the shunt dependency because these patients had had slit ventricles on the CAT scans prior to death. The definition of a slit ventricle is: on CAT scan, ventricles appear as a slit-like Y-shape and the ventricular space for the drainage of cerebrospinal fluid apparently becomes extremely slim. The subarachnoid space is never wide open as it is in the case of so-called cerebral atrophy or similar conditions (fig. 1).

How often does slit ventricle occur (table II)? Well over one third of those patients who had ventriculoperitoneal shunts and follow-up CAT scans showed slit ventricle. Those suffering from slit ventricle would have died due to shunt obstruction without careful monitoring.

Table I. What group of hydrocephalus?

Type of hydrocephalus	Number of survivors	Number of deaths	Total in group
Congenital	27	1	28
Spina bifida-associated	37	3	40
Post-infective	21	1	22
Acquired non-infective	16	0	16
Total	101	5	106

All cases had repeated CAT scans. More than 12 months follow-up.

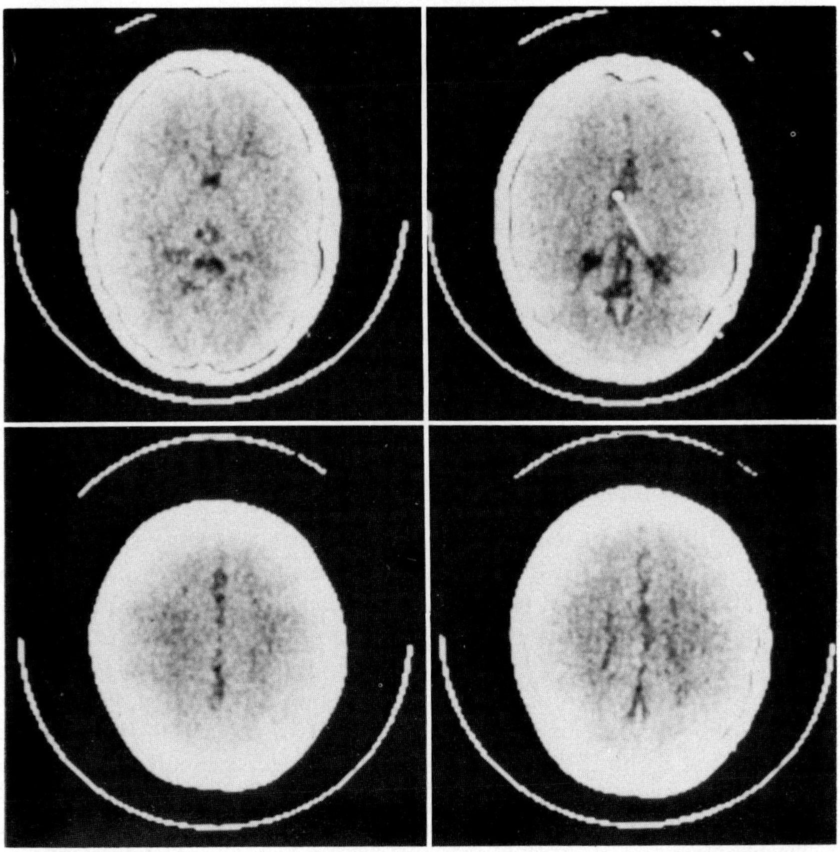

Fig. 1. CAT scan of a 5-year-old girl 4 years after ventriculoperitoneal shunt operation. An example of a slit ventricle.

Table II. How often does slit ventricle occur?

Type of hydrocephalus	Number of survivors	Number of slit ventricles	% in group
Congenital	27	8	29
Spina bifida-associated	37	16	43
Post-infective	21	7	33
Acquired non-infective	16	4	25
Total	101	35	

Table III. How serious is a slit ventricle?

Handicap		Number of cases (%)	% from Laurence's natural history	Number of slit ventricles (% in group)
mental	physical			
Normal	normal	24		12 (50)
	slightly	5 (31)	18	2
	severely	2		1
	incapacitated	0		0
Subnormal	normal	4		1
	slightly	7		1
	severely	4 (16)	16	2
Ineducable		37		15 (40)
Death		(5)	49	5
Total		106		40

How were they evaluated? Because of the tremendous variety in the development during childhood, we found the classification by Laurence to be most agreeable. Distribution of the IQ test is accommodated in between each group.

How serious is a slit ventricle (table III)? In comparison with the follow-up results of the non-shunted group by Laurence, we can see a brilliant success achieved by ventriculoperitoneal shunts in reduction of mortality; however, on the other hand, at least one half of the patient who escaped death become ineducable. That is the first point from this result and, secondly, a goal of the ventriculoperitoneal shunts can be the slit ventricle because the slit ventricle was found almost exclusively in either normal or ineducable groups. Naturally, this is only apparent when we concentrate on the statistical points only and neglect the clinical history of each patient.

In conclusion, this study confirmed the impression that a slit ventricle is the reluctant but ultimate goal of a functioning ventriculoperitoneal shunt rather than a simple complication which was found in a small portion of shunted children. In view of this result and too many serious complications (infection and obstruction), the author feels that the period of ventriculoperitoneal shunt has passed and a new method, such as 'microsurgical suprapineal ventriculostomy', ought to be developed by the author for the next generation.

A. Hirayama, MD, Kobe University School of Medicine, 12 Kusunoki-cho 7-chome, Ikuta-ku, Kobe (Japan)

Monogr. neural Sci., vol. 8, pp. 112–116 (Karger, Basel 1982)

Intracranial Pressure Patterns in the Shunt-Dependent Hydrocephalus

P.L. Longatti, M.A. Gerosa, A. Olivi, A. Carteri

Istituto di Neurochirurgia (Director: Prof. *P. Frugoni*), Sezione di Neurochirurgia Infantile (Associated Prof.: Prof. *A. Carteri*), Università degli Studi di Padova, Padova, Italy

Introduction

It is not easy to give an all-inclusive definition of shunt-independent hydrocephalus (SIH); with approximation we could define it as a condition of treated hydrocephalus in which the shunt could be removed without further increase of ventricular dilatation and with stabilized intracranial pressure values. Previous reports analyzed the occurrence of SIH in children who at control showed an asymptomatic obstruction of their shunts [1–3]. In this paper we review our experience about SIH in a group of 41 children with well-functioning shunts.

Materials and Methods

41 treated hydrocephalic children were examined; their ages ranged from 7 months to 10 years. In table I the etiology of the hydrocephalus is summarized. All the patients had placed a medium pressure multipurpose valve (MPV) provided by an on-off control mechanism allowing the opening and the closing of the shunt. The time elapsed from the first shunting procedure was between 2 and 5 years.

The patency of the shunt was ascertained through a global judgment based on: pumping maneuvres, intracranial pressure (ICP) monitoring, and different pressure saline infusion of the peritoneal catheter. The first time the working pressure was monitored through the MPV reservoir. After 60 min the CSF flow was interrupted pushing the on-off control into shutting position. The test was stopped when the ICP increased indefinitely or when an 'A wave' appeared or clinical signs of intracranial hypertension occurred. 15 children were submitted to CT scan and Evan's index, i.e. the frontal horn ratio, was derived.

Results

37 of 41 tested children developed pathological intracranial pressure. We define 'latency time' (LT) as the time elapsed between the moment of the MPV

Table I. Types of hydrocephalus

	Number
Communicating	
Congenital	6
Postmeningitic	8
Posthemorrhagic	2
Unknown	7
Blocked	
Aqueduct stenosis	5
Decompensation wave	4
Meningomyelocele	5
Tumoral	4
	41

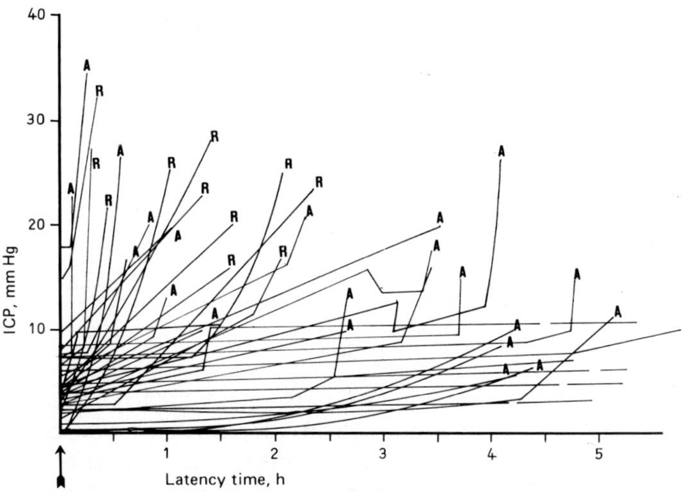

Fig. 1. Arrow indicates the working pressure of the shunt. A = Plateau waves; R = ramp waves.

shutting and the first manifest decompensation pressure wave. In this series the LT varied from 5 min to 7 h; however, in about 75% it was limited to 1 h (fig. 1). Although all the patients showed a patent shunt, in 2 cases a working pressure of the valve higher than 10 mm Hg and a related short LT was demonstrated. The most usual ICP patterns are diagrammatically reported in figure 2.

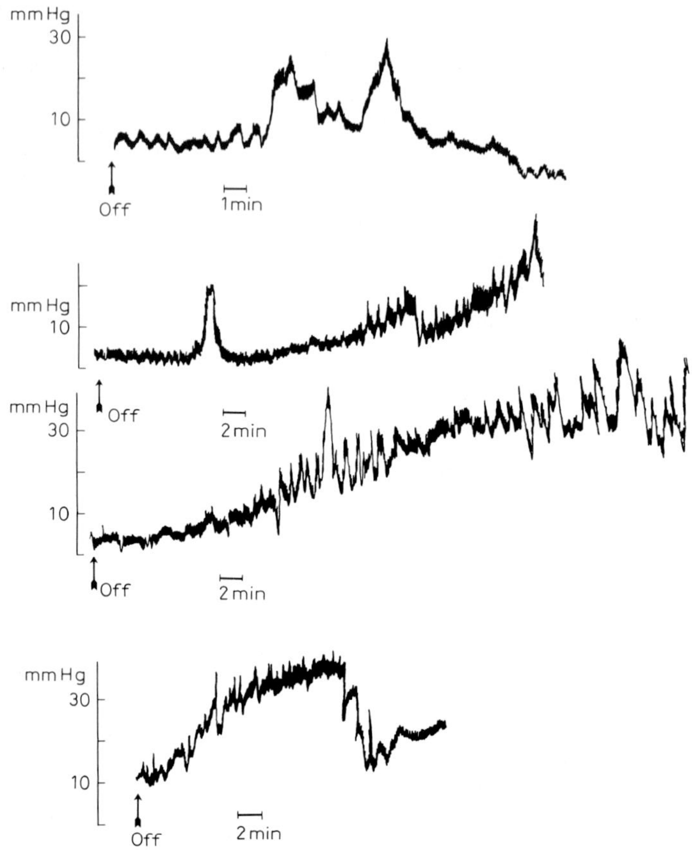

2a

Fig. 2. a Examples of ICP tracing. *b* The decompensation hypertensive wave is indicated by a curved arrow.

4 cases who manifested a persistent flat tracing over 8 h of monitoring belonged to the group of tumoral hydrocephalus (3 cerebellar astrocytomas and 1 medulloblastoma) operated almost 1 year before. These patients could be regarded as control cases. The relation between the frontal horn ratio and LT seems evident only for the cases with an opening pressure of less than 7.5 mm Hg (fig. 3).

Discussion

It is generally accepted that the surgically treated hydrocephalus becomes shunt-independent when the shunt is not patent, the ICP is found within normal

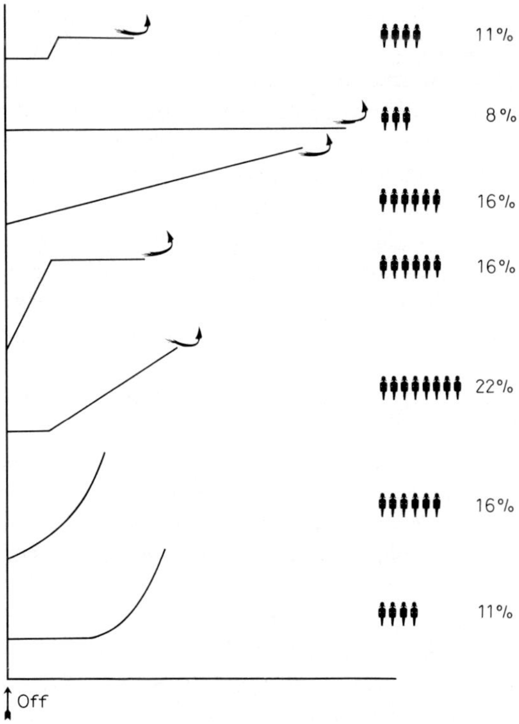

2b

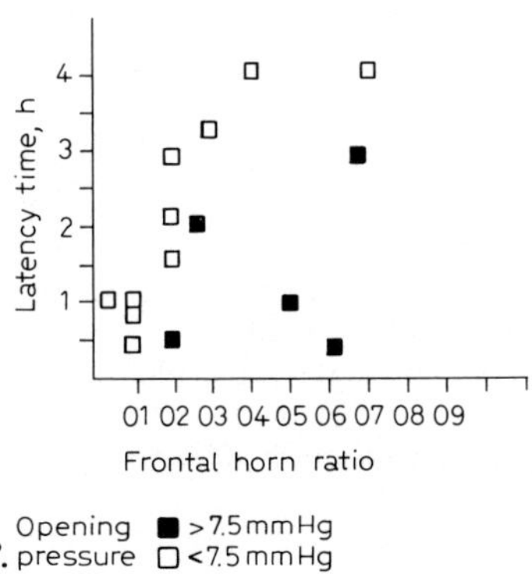

Fig. 3.

ranges and a further ventricular enlargement can be excluded. If these conditions are not accomplished it is difficult to discriminate the SIH from other situations as the mild hypertension hydrocephalus, the intermittent hypertension hydrocephalus and even the normal pressure hydrocephalus.

The occurrence of SIH is still debated in the literature [1–3]. *Holtzer et al.* [3] screened 34 out of 126 treated hydrocephalic children whose shunt was found spontaneously occluded and normal ICP values with stabilized ventricular enlargement were assessed. It is impressive to observe that in about 25 % of these cases the ventricle size evaluated by two-dimensional echoencephalography showed normal values although the reliability of this method could be questioned. Furthermore, methodologic details regarding the evaluation of ICP are not fully specified and that seems not negligible since the differential diagnosis of SIF from other conditions (see above) needs a long-standing monitoring of ICP and infusion tests. In our study all the patients manifested hypertensive ICP tracing after the shutting of MPV and that seems to exclude the occurrence of SIH.

Probably the CSF physiologically produced first accumulated without determining an increase of ICP. The duration of this phase depends upon the working pressure of the shunt, the ventricular enlargement, and the compliance of the system. Thereafter, the ICP rises linearly or exponentially, and then a decompensation wave ensues (fig. 1). Sometimes the intracranial hypertension develops with subsequent stabilized plateaux indicating a further balance in CSF absorption– soon achieved but very soon lost.

It is very impressive to observe the great variability of the slope, morphology, and LT of these ICP tracings. This means that a different degree of shunt dependence is evident in every patient. The correlation between the LT and the ventricular size (fig. 3) is influenced by the working pressure of the shunt.

The test, as we performed, could be regarded as an autoinfusion of the CSF physiologically produced by the patient and temporarily not more diversioned by the shunt; the reliability of this method is comparable to the infusion tests.

References

1 Epstein, F.; Hochwald, G.; Ranshohoff, J.: Avoidance of shunt dependency in hydrocephalus. Devl Med. Child Neur. *17:* suppl. 35, pp. 71–77 (1975).

2 Foltz, E.L.; Shutleff, D.B.: Five years comparative study of hydrocephalus in children with and without operation (113 cases). J. Neurosurg. *20:* 1064–1079 (1963).

3 Holtzer, G.; Lange, Samuel A. de: Shunt-independent arrest of hydrocephalus. J. Neurosurg. *39:* 698–701 (1973).

Dr. P.L. Longatti, Istituto di Neurochirurgia dell'Università di Padova, Policlinico, I–35100 Padova (Italy)

Monogr. neural Sci., vol. 8, pp. 117–119 (Karger, Basel 1982)

Shunt Dependency in Myelomeningocele

C. Di Rocco
Istituto di Neurochirurgia, Università Cattolica, Roma, Italy

Owing to longer survival and improved postoperative conditions in a large number of operated on hydrocephalic children the neurosurgeon is often requested by patient's parents to remove the inserted CSF shunt assembly. The present report outlines some findings obtained when evaluating children, with hydrocephalus secondary to myelomeningocele, who had been considered for the possible removal of the CSF shunt device on the basis of a benign postoperative clinical evolution.

Material and Methods

7 children, of both sexes and ranging in age from 3 to 7 years with hydrocephalus associated to myelomeningocele were evaluated. 3 of them had been operated on in the first weeks of life and were given a ventriculo-atrial (VA) CSF shunt. They had been proposed among a larger group of patients for the possible removal of the inserted CSF device on the basis of a positive postoperative clinical history, the absence of CSF shunt revisions in the last 5 years, and the apparent upward migration of the distal end of the VA shunt into the jugular vein as seen by chest X-ray control. For checking the CSF shunt patency a telethermographic examination was performed in these 3 subjects [2]. The remaining 4 children had been admitted for evaluation because of mild psychomotor retardation. In all of them the hydrocephalus, noticed in the first months of life, was considered 'arrested'. A CT scan for evaluating the size and morphology of the ventricular system and a spinal subarachnoid infusion test (IT) for studying the CSF absorption [1] were carried out in this group of patients.

Results

Telethermography. In all the 3 children examined a CSF flow within the shunt assembly was detected by the characteristic linear precocious rewarming of the skin above the distal catheter.

CT Scan. Two main types of ventricular dilatation were observed. Type one (2 cases) was characterized by a homogeneous ventricular enlargement, which apparently was depending on the stenosis of the aqueduct; the ventricular walls were smooth. In type two (2 cases), the hydrocephalus was accompanied by a Chiari II malformation. The ventricular dilatation was mostly evident at the occipital horns and the ventricular contours were irregular.

IT. While in the first type hydrocephalus, the spinal infusion tests gave results comparable to those obtained in children with simple aqueductal stenosis, i.e. a progressive increase in the CSF pressure during the infusion until a plateau, in the second type hydrocephalus a characteristic biphasic response was obtained. In fact, the rapid increase in intracranial pressure in the first phase of the test was followed by a late return towards the normal values.

Discussion and Conclusions

Hydrocephalus associated with myelomeningocele exhibits several often noted and puzzling features: (1) although ventricular dilatation is almost certainly present in utero and at birth in infants who later develop clinical signs of progressive hydrocephalus, at the time of birth signs of hypertensive progressive hydrocephalus are usually lacking; (2) even when an abnormal increase in head circumference takes place, the signs of intracranial hypertension may remain lacking or they may be of a relatively mild degree; (3) finally, when ventricular dilatation with an increase in head circumference obviously occurs, the rate of its progression in the single subject may vary in time; furthermore, in most children transitory phases of an apparent 'arrest' of the syndrome are not infrequent. Such features have brought some authors, especially those concerned with pediatric practice, to regard the hydrocephalus associated with myelomeningocele as relatively benign in nature; in other words, to the erroneous belief that a spontaneous arrest of the ventricular dilatation may occur in a large number of cases. On the grounds of such an attitude, a hope is often generated in parents of operated on children that it might be possible to remove the inserted CSF shunt device.

In our experience, this hope is often unjustified. In fact, in the last few years, the wider use of techniques for investigating CSF dynamics has demonstrated the large incidence of slow evolving hydrocephalus in patients clinically regarded as affected by stabilized hydrocephalus [1, 3]. In this group of patients were included children with myelomeningocele whose associated hydrocephalus had not been treated [1].

Telethermographic evaluation in our 3 children with myelomeningocele and hydrocephalus operated on at birth demonstrated the patency of the CSF shunt inserted many years before. These children had been considered for the possible removal of their shunt on the basis of upward migration of the distal end of the VA shunt into the jugular vein and a history of no shunt revision in the last 5 years. Particularly interesting are the findings provided by the IT, namely the characteristic biphasic response observed in the children with Chiari type II malformation. In fact, according to this result, in some hydrocephalic children with myelomeningocele, the low-pressure range absorption mechanisms are defective, while those acting at the high-pressure levels are normal. In these patients the progression of the hydrocephalus may be particularly insidious, as obvious intracranial hypertensive states can hardly occur. Consequently, the same children may show an apparent 'arrest' of the hydrocephalus.

The insertion of a CSF shunt device theoretically might curtail this kind of compensatory mechanism, thus explaining the shunt dependency which was found at the telethermographic evaluation in all of our examined children.

In our opinion, such a possibility should suggest great caution in planning the removal of an inserted CSF shunt device in children treated for hydrocephalus associated with myelomeningocele, when the latter is accompanied by Chiari type II malformation.

References

1 Caldarelli, M.; Di Rocco, C.; Rossi, G.F.: Lumbar subarachnoid infusion test in paediatric neurosurgical practice. Devl Med. Child Neurol *21:* 71–82 (1979).

2 De Santis, M.; Caldarelli, M.; Cellini, N.; Di Rocco, C.: Telethermographic method for detecting CSF shunt patency in children. Rays *4:* 101–107 (1979).

3 Di Rocco, C.; Caldarelli, M.; Maira, G.; Rossi, G.F.: The study of CSF dynamics in apparently arrested hydrocephalus in children. Child's Brain *3:* 359–374 (1977).

C. Di Rocco, MD, Istituto di Neurochirurgia, Università Cattolica – Policlinico Gemelli, Largo Gemelli 8, I–00168 Roma (Italy)

Monogr. neural Sci., vol. 8, pp. 120–121 (Karger, Basel 1982)

CSF Shunt and the Electroencephalogram

H. Gastaut, N. Pinsard
Hôpital de la Timone, Marseille, France

The EEG is of little interest in the positive diagnosis of hydrocephalus since the anomalies found on EEG are most often related to the causative lesion and not the hydrocephalus itself. The only example of the diagnostic usefulness of EEG is the special case where hydrocephalus is so pronounced that the walls of the cerebral hemispheres lie flattened against and adherent to the cranial vault, in which case the distinction between brain matter and cranial bone is not revealed by computerized tomography (CT). In such cases, CT data may be suggestive of hydranencephaly. Consequently, EEG is of considerable diagnostic aid as no electrical activity is found in cases of hydranencephaly, whereas cortical activity persists even in extreme cases of hydrocephalus.

Conversely, EEG is of major importance to monitor the course of hydrocephalus treated by shunt. In this respect, focal polymorphous delta waves are recorded in the region surrounding the valve implant site in more than 50% of cases. These EEG signs may be present by the first few postoperative days, decreasing thereafter in some cases, or may be found to progress during the months after surgery.

EEG signs of irritation (spikes and spike waves) develop later on in the region of the implant site in 33–65% of cases, according to authors (a reasonable estimate would be about 50% of cases). Approximately 80% of such patients develop epileptic seizures, in agreement with an overall frequency of epilepsy in 25–50% of children having undergone a shunting procedure. The epileptic seizures usually occur months or years after the onset of the EEG abnormalities. Although diverse types of epilepsy can be found, the most frequent seizures are minor motor seizures of the Lennox-Gastaut syndrome and partial or hemiclonic seizures on the side opposite the EEG abnormalities. The occurrence of hemiclonic status epilepticus leading to hemiplegia has been observed, thus indicating the necessity to institute anticonvulsive therapy at the onset of signs of irritation or even earlier, when focal delta activity persists.

Finally, it should be pointed out that EEG abnormalities, especially those of an epileptic nature (and the resulting seizures), often undergo aggravation in cases where the shunt functions poorly or intracranial pressure increases. In conclusion, these data indicate that EEG is a particularly useful procedure in the follow-up of the course of hydrocephalus in children with a CSF shunt.

H. Gastaut, MD, Hôpital de la Timone, Rue Saint Pierre;
F–13005 Marseille (France)

Monogr. neural Sci., vol. 8, pp. 122–124 (Karger, Basel 1982)

The Abnormal Electroencephalogram and Epileptic Seizures in Children with Hydrocephalus

Juliusz Wocjan, Halina Wocjan, Krzysztof Wocjan
Child's Health Center, Department of Pediatric Neurosurgery
(Head: *Juliusz Wocjan*), Warszawa, Poland

The treatment of hydrocephalus presents many clinical problems and questions, not only in etiology, diagnostic and type of operative procedure but also in the occurring of various complications.

One of these complications – the incidence of epileptic seizures and EEG abnormalities after the shunt operations – needs discussion because of rare presentation of such cases.

Case Material

Our experience is based on clinical observations of 60 cases of hydrocephalic children, treated in the Department of Pediatric Neurosurgery (Warsaw, Poland), during the last 9 years. These cases were found among 493 children operated following symptoms of hydrocephalus caused by different etiological factors. In this presentation we included only cases of hydrocephalus caused by inflammatory process (hemorrhage or infection; 49 cases) or undetermined lesion (11 cases). The presented group consists of children surviving operation and observed from 2 to 8 years, in whom the EEG records were performed before the operation and at least once a year after the operation. We assumed that in other types of hydrocephalus (as caused by intracranial tumors, congenital malformations of the occipitocervical region or aqueductal stenosis) other factors could be responsible for EEG abnormalities independently of shunt operation.

The age of patients ranged between 6 weeks and 6 years. In all children we performed routine diagnostic procedures as ventriculography or angiography and in some cases CT scan. All children were operated upon using a Pudenz-Heyer valve.

Before the operative procedure the epileptic seizures were present in 8 cases (5 patients aged under 1 year): in 3 cases focal epilepsy and in 5 cases generalized seizures. After the shunt operation the epileptic seizures were observed in 28 children (in 18 under 1 year). Left-sided focal motor seizures were most common in children with right-sided shunts and were stated in 22 cases. In the remaining 6 cases general seizures were present.

Before the operation the abnormal electroencephalogram was observed in 50 of 52 children without epilepsy and in all epileptic patients. In patients without epilepsy the most

Table I. Type of EEG changes in 60 hydrocephalic children

	Before operation					After operation			
	No. of cases	generalized changes	epileptogenic focus	interhemispheric asymmetry	normal	No. of cases	generalized changes	epileptogenic focus	interhemispheric asymmetry
Without epileptic seizures	52	29	4	17	2	32	3	17	12
Epileptic seizures	8	–	3	5	–	28	2	22	4
Total	60	29	7	22	2	60	5	39	16

common finding presented generalized changes (delta-theta activity) or interhemispheric asymmetry. In children with epileptic fits in 3 cases epileptogenic focus was observed and in 5 cases interhemispheric asymmetry (table I).

After the shunting procedure the incidence of EEG changes was observed in all children. An epileptogenic focus was developed in 39 children (22 patients with seizures and 17 without epilepsy). In 16 cases interhemispheric asymmetry with the predominance over the shunted hemisphere was observed (4 cases with epilepsy and 12 cases without seizures). In the remaining cases generalized changes were stated.

All these irritative abnormalities started during the first year after the operative procedure and were seen during the entire period of observation. The epileptic seizures were stated in the postoperative period, beginning from 1 week to 10 months after the operation. In 7 cases, after administration of anticonvulsive therapy, the seizures withdrew.

Discussion and Conclusions

Discussing our clinical material we can consider that postoperative EEG changes and epileptic seizures present serious problems not so often presented because of the prevalence of other severe postoperative complications. The appearance of a brain lesion is caused following development and increase of intracranial hypertension by activating a chain of harmful events often of the 'vicious circle' type. According to the individual characteristics of the patient – his age, the state of his circulatory and respiratory system – and to the nature and localization of the brain lesion (all these factors conditioning the dynamics and mechanism of the forming intracranial hypertension), various components of intracranial contents contribute in different ways to the course of the developing events. In some cases there is time and space for compensatory possibilities to develop. This compensation however is not unlimited of course;

most often all intracranial elements contribute to some extent to aggravate the situation caused by hydrocephalus.

The incidence of EEG abnormalities over the shunted hemisphere and their localization – in the neighborhood of the shunt – can suggest that the valve may act as an irritative factor and could be responsible at least in part for observed EEG changes as well as for epileptic seizures. It is very probable that the age at the time of operation (the youngest group) can influence the occurrence of epilepsy. On the other hand the type of hydrocephalus and presence of preoperative brain lesion can be of importance in the development of epileptic seizures.

Juliusz Wocjan, MD, Mierosławskiego 24/1, PL–01–558 Warszawa (Poland)

Monogr. neural Sci., vol. 8, pp. 125–127 (Karger, Basel 1982)

Influences of Intracranial Pressure on Epileptic Activity

M. Caldarelli, C. Di Rocco, A. Iannelli
Istituto di Neurochirurgia, Università Cattolica, Roma, Italia

Clinical observation suggests that in some hydrocephalic children the EEG tracings may deteriorate when the CSF shunt assembly is not properly working. The aim of the present report is to describe the effects of increases in intracranial pressure (ICP) on experimentally induced epilepsy in animals.

Material and Methods

For the study 22 adult rabbits were utilized. Cortical or hippocampal epileptogenic foci were created with a topical application of penicillin. To raise the intracranial pressure, saline was infused at a constant rate (0.17 ml/min) for 10 min within the lumbar subarachnoid space; a Y connector allowed the continuous recording of intracranial pressure in the basal condition and during the infusion.

In 4 'cortical' animals and in 3 'hippocampal' animals a second experimental session was performed the day following the creation of the epileptogenic focus, after epilepsy disappeared.

Results

1. Basal Conditions

Prior to the creation of the epileptogenic focus, the artificially induced ICP increase did not produce any epileptic discharge; however, desynchronization of the EEG recording was always evident. On the other hand, the firing of the experimental focus modified the resting ICP values in only 1 animal.

2. Hippocampal Animals

In the 'hippocampal' rabbits, following the creation of the epileptogenic focus, the artificially induced ICP increase enhanced epileptic discharges during or soon after (few minutes) the first saline infusion (fig. 1).

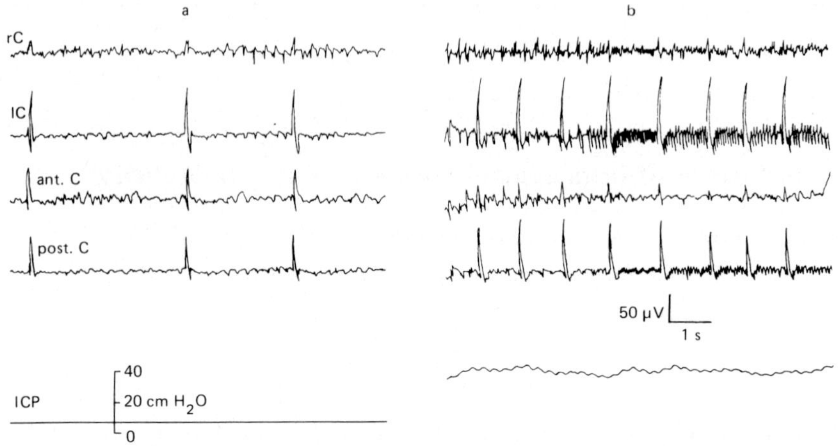

Fig. 1. a Basal EEG as in the text activity recorded from a left hippocampal focus. *b* Enhancement of the epileptic activity during saline infusion. rC = Right cortex; lC = left cortex; ant. C = anterior cortex; post. C = posterior cortex; ICP = intracranial pressure.

In 2 animals a decrease of epileptogenic activity and a depression of EEG tracings were recorded when high values of ICP (> 40 cm H_2O) were attained.

In the 3 animals in which the second experimental session was performed 24 h after epileptogenic focus creation, when the epileptic activity had disappeared, the renewal of epilepsy did not follow the artificial increases in ICP.

3. Cortical Animals

Enhancement of epileptogenic activity occurred in all the animals, following the increase in ICP. However, the finding was apparent only after the third infusion test. Generally, the phenomenon was better appreciated when the pressure values had almost returned within the resting limits, but in 1 rabbit the enhancement was apparent already during the infusion.

In the 4 animals investigated the day following the epileptogenic focus creation, the epilepsy had spontaneously subsided. In all of them the renewal of focus activity was obtained. Again it was necessary to perform three saline infusions before recording the phenomenon.

Discussion and Conclusions

The clinical translation of experimental findings in humans is always hard. Species differences as well as different modalities of creation and organization of the epileptic activity should be taken into account when trying to utilize our experimental data in clinical practice. However, the overview of our results seems to indicate that a relationship between epileptic activity and variations in ICP occurs in most instances. Such a statement is supported by the occurrence of the enhancement of the basal epileptic activity when increases in ICP are induced as well as by the renewal of an apparently cleared epileptogenic focus.

These findings, which correspond to clinical observations, stress the importance of EEG monitoring in the postoperative evaluation of operated hydrocephalic epileptic children. However, the physiopathogenic interpretation of the above-mentioned relationship between epilepsy and variations in ICP remains obscure. Indeed, significant differences in the response to the ICP increases were recorded depending on the anatomical location of the epileptogenic lesions. Furthermore, the enhancement in the epileptic activity did not follow the increases in ICP immediately; it could persist even when ICP had returned to normal limits.

M. Caldarelli, MD, Istituto di Neurochirurgia, Università Cattolica, I–00168 Roma (Italia)

Monogr. neural Sci., vol. 8, pp. 128–129 (Karger, Basel 1982)

EEG Systematic Controls of Shunted Hydrocephalic Children

A. Beaumanoir, J. Berney

Laboratoire d'EEG du Département de Neurologie, Clinique Universitaire de Pédiatrie, Clinique Universitaire de Neurochirurgie, Genève, Suisse

29 hydrocephalic children, treated with a Spitz-Holter ventriculo-atrial shunt, have been followed electroclinically for at least 8 years. 19 among them developed spikes in their EEG at the site of the first operation within 5 years (fig. 1), they all had at least one postoperative seizure and 17 had to be treated with anticonvulsive drugs. 5 children had a severe epilepsy. This was the situation 5 years after the first shunt (fig. 2) [1].

In 1980 there are still 26 cases under control. 1 patient died and 2 are lost. The 7 children with a normal EEG still have a normal EEG. Of the 5 children who were considered to have a severe epilepsy, 1 is lost (neonatal cerebral hemorrhage), 3 are still very difficult to treat, 1 cannot be considered anymore to have a severe epilepsy, but is treated. 17 children had to be treated to prevent the occurrence of fits, 14 are still under treatment, 1 is no more treated and 2 are lost. 1 child had a focal seizure, who did not have before. Thus, the situation has not changed very much, but has certainly not deteriorated.

The disease underlying the hydrocephalus seems to be responsible for the development of an epilepsy which must be treated, but the focus of spikes is certainly related to the insertion of the valve and can trigger the occurrence of focal seizures.

The cases related to neonatal hemorrhage appear to have a very high risk of epilepsy. On the contrary this risk in the myelomeningoceles is low. In this group one of the two treated children had meningitis before 6 months of age, whilst in the second there is no explanation except the valve for the development of the irritative focus, which is present in the EEG of both.

In the other cases the necessity for a treatment with anticonvulsant drugs can be concomitant with the presence of a cerebral focal deficit (4/10 cases). But what is striking in all the cases is the frequency of the irritative focus which is always under the valve, and the focal caracter of the seizures.

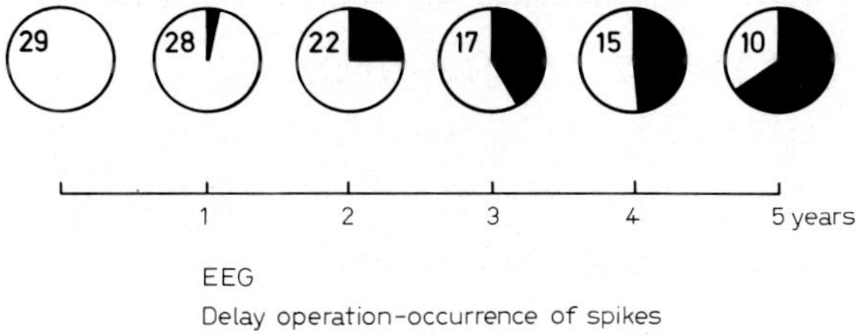

Fig. 1. The time course of the appearance of focal spikes on successive EEG recordings.

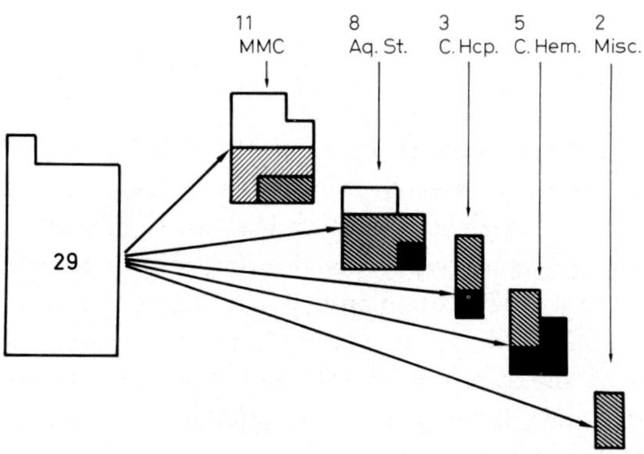

Fig. 2. The electroclinical evolution of the 29 children, divided according to the etiology of the hydrocephalus (1977). Each square represent 1 child. Black square = severe epilepsy; dark gray square = treated epilepsy; light gray square = at least one fit; white square = no fit at all. MMC = Myelomeningocele; Aq.St. = aqueduct stenosis; C. Hcp. = communicating hydrocephalus; C. Hem. = neonatal cerebral hemorrhage; Misc. = 1 neonatal subdural hematoma, 1 complex malformation.

Reference

1 Varfis, G.; Berney, J.; Beaumanoir, A.: Electro-clinical follow-up of shunted hydrocephalic children. Child's Brain *3:* 129–139 (1977).

A. Beaumanoir, MD, Laboratoire d'EEG du Département de Neurologie, Clinique Universitaire de Pédiatrie, Clinique Universitaire de Neurochirurgie,
CH–1200 Genève (Suisse)

Monogr. neural Sci., vol. 8, pp. 130–133 (Karger, Basel 1982)

Outcome in Shunted Hydrocephalic Patients[1]

Howard M. Eisenberg, Maryann Thompson, Harvey S. Levin

Division of Neurosurgery, Department of Surgery, The University of Texas Medical Branch, Galveston, Tex., USA

The observation that cognitive outcome in children with hydrocephalus after shunting is not uniform has led to research into factors which may account for this variability. The etiology of hydrocephalus appears to be important, in that children who have uncomplicated hydrocephalus fare better than those whose hydrocephalus is associated with brain injury [6]. Cognitive outcome with myelomeningocele is less clear [4, 5]. In many studies it appears that, at least in infants, the width of the cerebral mantle prior to shunting is not associated with cognitive outcome; however, a thin mantle after shunting is generally associated with cognitive deficit [2, 6].

Several studies have investigated specific cognitive and perceptual deficits [3] but these studies do not relate the deficits to etiology or computed tomographic (CT) findings. In the present study, we have evaluated treated hydrocephalic children with concurrent neuropsychological tests and CT scans.

Clinical Material

We have studied 63 children. No etiology was excluded except brain tumor. The median age at the time of evaluation was 3.3 years (range 3 months to 13.9 years). There were 33 girls and 30 boys. All social classes were represented; approximately 70% were from the working class or lower. Median age at the time of the first shunt operation was 2.4 months (range 0.5–14 months), with all but 20% of the children receiving the first shunt by the age of 6 months.

[1] This study was supported by the March of Dimes Birth Defects Foundation Clinical Research Grant No. 6–173.

Methods

The patients' histories were reviewed without reference to the psychological testing or the CT scan for evidence of primary brain injury apart from hydrocephalus (e.g. infection or hemorrhage) that occurred before or after the insertion of the shunt. Cases considered to have brain injury other than hydrocephalus were termed 'complicated hydrocephalus'; if there was no evidence of such an event and a patient's hydrocephalus appeared to be the result of a congenital anomaly, the case was termed 'uncomplicated'.

Each child received a general test of mental ability: a standard intelligence test (yielding an IQ) for children over 2½ years or the Bayley Scales of Infant Development (yielding a developmental quotient, DQ) for younger children. We assigned a mental quotient of 40 to patients whose scores were too low to be read from the test tables. Children over the age of 2½ additionally received language and visuospatial-visuomotor tests. Each child's CT scan was examined and the view which best displayed the lateral ventricles was selected. The intracranial contents and the lateral ventricles were measured with a polar compensating planimeter and the ventricle:brain ratio (VBR) was computed.

Results

Of the patients with complicated hydrocephalus (table I), approximately half were functioning in the range of mental retardation (IQ or DQ <70). Complicated patients with porencephaly fared worst of all; the highest mental quotient in that subgroup was 71. Uncomplicated patients had a better outcome, although mental retardation did appear here also. The difference in mental quotient between the complicated and uncomplicated groups yielded a significant Mann-Whitney U test ($p < 0.001$). Complicated cases with porencephaly had mental quotients significantly below each of the remaining groups ($p < 0.01$). Children with complicated hydrocephalus without porencephaly scored below the uncomplicated patients ($p < 0.01$). The difference between the two uncomplicated groups was not significant.

For children over the age of 2½ years, differences between the complicated and uncomplicated cases were compared in two specific areas. On the Peabody Picture Vocabulary Test, a measure of receptive vocabulary, the groups were significantly different ($p < 0.01$), with scores (medians 68.5 and 93.3) similar to the groups' mental quotients. The difference between the two groups was not significant on the Beery Test of Visual Motor Integration, a test of copying designs, with group medians (expressed as z-scores) of –2.4 for the complicated patients and –1.4 for the uncomplicated patients. Both these scores were less than the 10th percentile.

The median VBR of all patients was 11.8% (range 1–69%), compared to the normal VBR in children under 10 years old of 1.8% [1]. The complicated and uncomplicated groups did not differ in VBR. In uncomplicated patients there was a small correlation between VBR and mental quotient (IQ or DQ) which approach-

Table I. Distribution of mental quotient for the patient groups

	n	Median	Range
Complicated	35	69	40–113
With porencephaly	9	40.4	40–71
Without porencephaly[1]	26	70.5	40–113
Uncomplicated	25	90	40 -122
With myelomeningocele	13	90	79–122
Without myelomeningocele	12	87.5	40–109

[1] 3 patients omitted (2 were deaf, 1 did not cooperate for testing).

ed statistical significance ($\gamma = -0.22$, $p < 0.07$), i.e. for patients with uncomplicated hydrocephalus, a large VBR was associated with lower mental quotient. No similar relationship in the complicated groups was found.

We examined 45 patients a second time after 1 year. There was no change in mental quotient in that period, although there was a significant decrease in VBR in children under the age of 2½ years.

Discussion

Our study indicates that children with complicated hydrocephalus fare worse than those with uncomplicated hydrocephalus on tests of general intelligence and of receptive language; in these areas uncomplicated patients attain near normal scores. However, the majority of hydrocephalic children, regardless of etiology, do not have visuomotor skills commensurate with their overall cognitive ability. Our study also indicates that the presence of myelomeningocele is not a predictor of poor intellectual performance in treated hydrocephalic children. The relationship between mental quotient and VBR in uncomplicated patients is similar to that found by *Young et al.* [6]. This relationship may have clinical importance.

References

1 Barron, S.; Jacobs, L.; Kinkel, W.: Changes in size of normal lateral ventricles during aging determined by computerized tomography. Neurology, Minneap. *26:* 1011–1013 (1976).

2 Bottcher, J.; Jacobsen, S.; Gyldensted, C.; Harmsen, A.; Gloerselt-Tarp, B.: Intellectual development and brain size in 13 shunted hydrocephalic children. Neuropädiatrie *9:* 369–377 (1978).

3 Miller, E.; Sethi, L.: The effect of hydrocephalus on perception. Devl Med. Child Neurol. *13:* 77–81 (1971).

4 Raimondi, A.; Soare, P.: Intellectual development in shunted hydrocephalic children. Am. J. Dis. Child *127:* 664–671 (1974).

5 Tew, B.; Laurence, K.M.: The effect of hydrocephalus on intelligence, visual perception and school attainment. Devl Med. Child Neurol. *17:* suppl. 37, pp. 129–134 (1975).

6 Young, H.; Nulsen, F.; Weiss, M.; Thomas, P.: The relationship of intelligence and cerebral mantle in treated infantile hydrocephalus (IQ potential in hydrocephalic children). Pediatrics, Springfield *52:* 38–44 TX 77550 (USA)

H.M. Eisenberg, MD, Division of Neurosurgery, Department of Surgery, The University of Texas Medical Branch, Galveston, TX 77550 (USA)

Monogr. neural Sci., vol. 8, pp. 134–136 (Karger, Basel 1982)

Long-Term Assessment of Shunts in Hydrocephalus

John Lorber, Michael A. Reynolds
Department of Paediatrics, University of Sheffield, Sheffield, England

Introduction

It is frequently said that once a shunt has been inserted for the treatment of hydrocephalus that it needs to be a functioning shunt as long as the patient lives, if he is not to run into serious trouble. It is equally frequently said that a shunt which has been in position for many years without a revision ever having been carried out and which, of necessity, is anatomically in an unfavourable situation, cannot be functioning and need not function. A great many surgeons tell patients that their shunts are non-functioning. This may engender a false confidence, so that if and when shunt complications occur, they are attributed to other causes with grave danger to the patient's life and health.

Present Study

To resolve the problem we examined 167 individuals with hydrocephalus not due to tumour and not associated with spina bifida cystica or encephalocele, and who had a shunt inserted for at least 10 years and up to 21 years prior to the assessment (average 14 years). 7 are dead. Arbitrarily, the patients were divided into four catagories (table I).

Category 1 – Shunt no Longer Necessary: 28 patients (17%)
It was considered that patients no longer needed a shunt if the shunt was removed for any reason and not replaced within 2 years without clinical deterioration in the patient's condition and without additional enlargement of the ventricles. Patients were also considered not to need a shunt if X-rays and/or CT scans showed that the shunt has been detached or fragmented for at least 2 years or longer and who again showed no ill effects following the discovery of such detachment. As the patients are not X-rayed every year it is possible that some detachments, when discovered for the first time, have been present for many years. 28 patients fall into this category, being 17% of the total of 167.

Table I. Four categories of hydrocephalic patients

	Number	%
No need for shunt	28	17
1 If shunt removed without ill effect		
2 If shunt has been detached or disintegrated for years (X-ray, CT scan) without ill effect		
Shunt probably not needed	34	20
1 No revision for over 10 years		
and		
2 Distal catheter well out of heart (X-ray); very stiff		
or		
3 Proximal catheter out of lateral ventricle		
Shunt probably necessary	45	27
1 Revision(s) within past 8–10 years		
2 Shunt continous and in good position; compressible		
Shunt necessary	60	36
1 Revision(s) within 2 years, for clinical reason		
2 Shunt in good position		
3 Fatal shunt blockage		

Category 2 – Shunt Probably no Longer Necessary: 34 patients (20%)

The second category are patients who probably do not need a shunt. These never had a shunt revision or had no shunt revision for at least 10 years. Their shunts, therefore, on X-ray are usually anatomically in far from a favourable position. The scan may show that the tip of the ventricular catheter is either just within or not within the ventricle, and that the atrial catheter is well out of the heart, usually above the clavicle, but is continuous. The patient suffers no clinical symptoms suggestive of intracranial hypertension and has no such signs.

Nevertheless, at most some of these patients are still potentially at risk. There were several patients of that age group who would have belonged to this category but had major shunt problems occurring even 15 years after the last shunt revision and when they were already some 20 years of age. Ignoring the possibility of such events could have resulted in the death of such individuals, it did cause death in several who were already out of the care of the Sheffield Children's Hospital, whose typical symptoms were ignored. Some died at home, having been in good condition immediately prior to such an event.

Another example is one young man of 19½ who has not had a revision for over 10 years and had no symptoms of increased intracranial tension, and was in gainful occupation. Over a period of 2 days he developed acute headache with papilloedema. The lower catheter of the shunt was blocked; the tip of the catheter was in the superior vena cava. It was replaced by a peritoneal cathether with full recovery.

Category 3 – Shunt Probably Still Needed: 45 patients (27%)

The patients in this category are arbitrarily considered to be probably still in need of the shunt, because they had to have a revision for clinical reasons (not planned lengthening of tubes for prophylactic reasons) within 2–10 years prior to their assessment for this study. Their shunt is in continuity and they have no symptoms or signs of intracranial hypertension.

Category 4 – Shunt Definitely Needed: 60 patients (36%)

Finally, in category 4 are those who are considered to be definitely in need of a shunt, either because they had a revision for clinical reasons within the last 2 years of their last attendance, or died of shunt complications, irrespective of the time that the last revision occurred.

Discussion

It is clear from this study that there is an important proportion of individuals, at least 17%, who do manage to do without a shunt, having been dependent on it for a period prior to its removal or disintegration. The proportion of these is progressively increasing with increasing age and time between shunt insertion and years of follow-up. It is possible, therefore, that individuals who reached 20 years or more from shunt insertion are far less liable to be shunt-dependent than others. Accurate data on this cannot be obtained as yet.

Relatively few patients who had shunt insertion 20 or more years ago are yet alive. Further, it is difficult to secure full information about some, as they have left the Children's Hospital and often changed their addresses. It is difficult to obtain objective data about their condition.

Conclusion

It is concluded that it is only safe to assure patients or their relatives that the patient no longer needs a shunt if, in fact, he has not got one now or it is no longer in continuity and has been for over 2 years. The number in the second category will, no doubt, go into the first category as time goes on, but it is still wiser to regard them as potentially needing their shunt unless proved otherwise. Continued supervision of all such patients is essential.

Prof. J. Lorber, Department of Paediatrics, University of Sheffield,
Sheffield (England)

Monogr. neural Sci., vol. 8, pp. 137–139 (Karger, Basel 1982)

Precocious Puberty in Hydrocephalus

E. Paraicz, J. Örley, I. Gáti

National Institute of Neurosurgery and Postgraduate Medical School, Budapest, Hungary

Since the 1930s there has been a steady accumulation of data indicating precocious puberty in hydrocephalus [1–4]. Nowadays that intracranial hypertension can successfully be treated with CSF shunts, many of these patients have grown to reach the age of puberty. The pathological dynamic and cerebral blood flow factor, ischaemia, the enormous dilatation of the third ventricle and the massive thinning of its wall, etc., can be prevented. We are now faced with new problems to solve and difficulties to surmount in connection with the specific features of the hormone balance in these patients [5].

We have classified the 46 investigated patients into two groups. *Group I:* 8 boys and 5 girls with ventriculo-atrial shunt on account of progressive hydrocephalus, implanted during infancy. *Group II:* 17 boys and 16 girls who underwent surgery on account of myelodysplasia in the first or second 24 h of life. Of them 17 displayed significant clinical symptoms of hydrocephalus; 7 had ventriculo-atrial shunt implantation.

Examinations

Hormone Determinations are listed in table I.

Clinical Examination. Stature, skin fold, bone development (the genitalia and vaginal discharge).

Results

The results of hormone determinations are summarized in tables I and II. In group I, i.e. in the patients operated on due to infantile hydrocephalus, the luteinizing hormone values were elevated in both the girls and the boys, but only

Table I. Operated infantile hydrocephalus

Hormone	Boys		Girls	
	$\overline{X}$	SE	$\overline{X}$	SE
Follice-stimulating hormone, mU/ml	9.63	1.71	9.26	1.44
Luteinizing hormone, mU/ml	65.2	4.4	60.3	10.4
Human prolactin, ng/ml	12.4	0.7	13.1	0.61
Testosterone, ng/ml	0.92	0.1	–	–
Total oestrogen, μg/24 h	26.7	5.65	3.23	0.61
17-Ketosteroid, mg/24 h	2.25	0.1	3.43	1.49

Table II. Operated myelodysplasia and hydrocephalus

Hormone	Boys		Girls	
	$\overline{X}$	SE	$\overline{X}$	SE
Luteinizing hormone, mU/ml	24.3	3.85	6.96	0.23
Testosterone, ng/ml	1.54	0.09	–	–
Human prolactin, ng/ml	–	–	22.49	0.99

Table III. Early signs in girls

	Number of patients	Age, years
Precocious puberty	3	6, 8, 9
Precocious telarche	2	7, 7
Adrenarche	5	7, 7, 8, 8, 11
Premenarche	1	8
Secondary amenorrhoea	1	11
Postmenarche	2	9, 11
Total	14 (63.6%)	

the boys had a high total oestrogen level. In the spina bifida group the luteinizing hormone value of the boys was fourfold that of the girls, and the human prolactin value approached the upper normal limit also in the girls. Clinical examination disclosed marked signs of precocious puberty particularly in those patients in whom the shunt operation was associated with a high number of complications, such as meningitis, numerous shunt obstructions and, consequently, hypertensive conditions. The signs of precocious puberty were more obvious in girls (table III). Two girls have already passed menarche, two have pubertas praecox, and two telarche praecox. We ascribe the older bone age in the boys to the elevated testosterone level, because this could not be observed in the girls.

Our aim was to add some data to the accumulating information about the hormonal problems of puberty in patients with CSF shunt-treated hydrocephalus.

References

1 Thomas, A.; Schäffer, H.: Un cas de macrogénitosomie précoce avec hydrocéphalie, lésions inflammatoires de la région infundibulo-tuberienne et symphyse cervicale trimeningé sans néoplasme intracranienne. Revue neurol. *2:* 595 (1931).
2 Dorff, G.; Shapiro, L.: A clinicopathologic study of sexual precocity with hydrocephalus. Report of two cases occurring in females with postmortem observations in one. Am. J. Dis. Child. *53:* 481 (1937).
3 Jolly, H.: Female isosexual precocity. Clin. Obstet. Gynec. *3:* 197 (1960).
4 Fiedeleff, H.L.; Guidelman, A.; Mancini, A.M.; Debeljuk, L.; László, M.: Puberté précose vraie par hydrocéphalie congénitale. Exploration de l'axe hypothalamo-hypophyso-ovarienne. Nouv. Press méd. *4:* 2799 (1975).
5 Örley, J.; Gáti, I.; Paraicz, E.: Puberty in shunted infantile hydrocephalic cases. 4th Int. Symp. Pediatric Gynecology, Florence 1978 (in press).

E. Paraicz, MD, National Institute of Neurosurgery and Postgraduate Medical School, Budapest (Hungary)

Monogr. neural Sci., vol. 8, pp. 140–143 (Karger, Basel 1982)

Radiological Long-Term Follow-Up of Hydrocephalus

Charles Raybaud

Service de Neuro-Radiologie du Prof. *G. Salamon,* Hôpital de la Timone, Marseille, France

Hydrocephalus is a generic term describing a single pathological process (the active ventricular dilatation) that obeys to mechanisms which are often ill understood. It may be induced by numerous etiologies which are sometimes simple (obstructive tumoral hydrocephalus), and sometimes very complex. The active ventricular dilatation is related to disturbances of the CSF circulation, and also to a rupture of the forces of equilibrium between the CSF cavities and the brain tissue. To this ventricular dilatation, hydrocephalus may associate a neural difformity and curable or permanent histologic disorders. The generalized use of ventricular shunting, and the advent of CT scanning, have revealed that the ventricular pressure was only a part of the problem, the other part, the cerebral response, being actually the most significant. This response indicates the condition of the brain, the lesions of which may be the cause, the effect, or both, of hydrocephalus, or even simply associated to it (fig. 1).

Hydrocephalus itself may have a puzzling behavior. It is related not only to the circulation of CSF, but also to the force the CSF pressure applies on the walls of the CSF-containing cavities, and this force is related to the wall area of the cavities. All these facts explain why the morphology of hydrocephalus does not always respond simply to the ventricular drainage, and why long-term follow-up of the patients may be surprising.

Radiological follow-up has been made easy by CT scanning. What should be primarily looked for is the possibility of adverse effects of shunting. These include the development of subdural collections, the collapse of the ventricles, and an imbalance between the intracranial fluid cavities. Subdural collections indicate that the cerebral mantle compliance is lost, and that no improvement can be expected from a functional point of view. Ventricular collapse raises the risk of acute ventricular hypertension. Both these complications are due to a poorly adapted ventricular drainage. Imbalance between different fluid cavities may be encountered in brain malformations or brain cavitations, and in quadri-

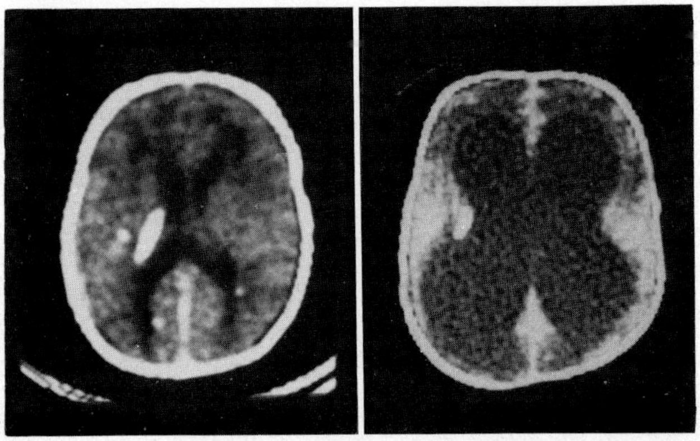

Fig. 1. *a* 1-month-old girl with toxoplasmosis. The ventricles are hardly enlarged. Beside the calcifications, the CT scan reveals a low density of the frontal white matter. *b* Same case, 2.5 months later: the ventricles are markedly enlarged, and the frontal low-density area indicates the permanent parenchymal damage, and not a reversible CSF transependymal egress.

Table I. Morphological results after ventricular drainage (127 cases)

	Satisfactory, %	Poor, %
Tumoral hydrocephalus	100	
Myelomeningocele	65	35
Other brain malformations	42	58
Perinatal hemorrhage	43	57
Postinfectious hydrocephalus	35	65

ventricular hydrocephalus. It necessitates to be alleviated by multiple shunting, with the risk of further imbalance.

On the whole, the radiological point of view on chronic hydrocephalus is rather pessimistic. A survey of 127 cases made in our institution reveals that beside the tumoral hydrocephalus and, to a lesser degree, hydrocephalus associated with myelomeningoceles, the morphological results are poor in more than half the cases (table I). Moreover, there is no real correlation between the morphological result and the functional result, the latter not being usually really improved. On the other hand, the neurological symptoms related to hydrocephalus are usually relieved by shunting, and any recurrence of symptoms is usually related to dysfunctioning of the drainage material. This leads to the practical attitude concerning the follow-up of shunted patients. Except for the few months following the shunt placement, when CT examination evaluates the

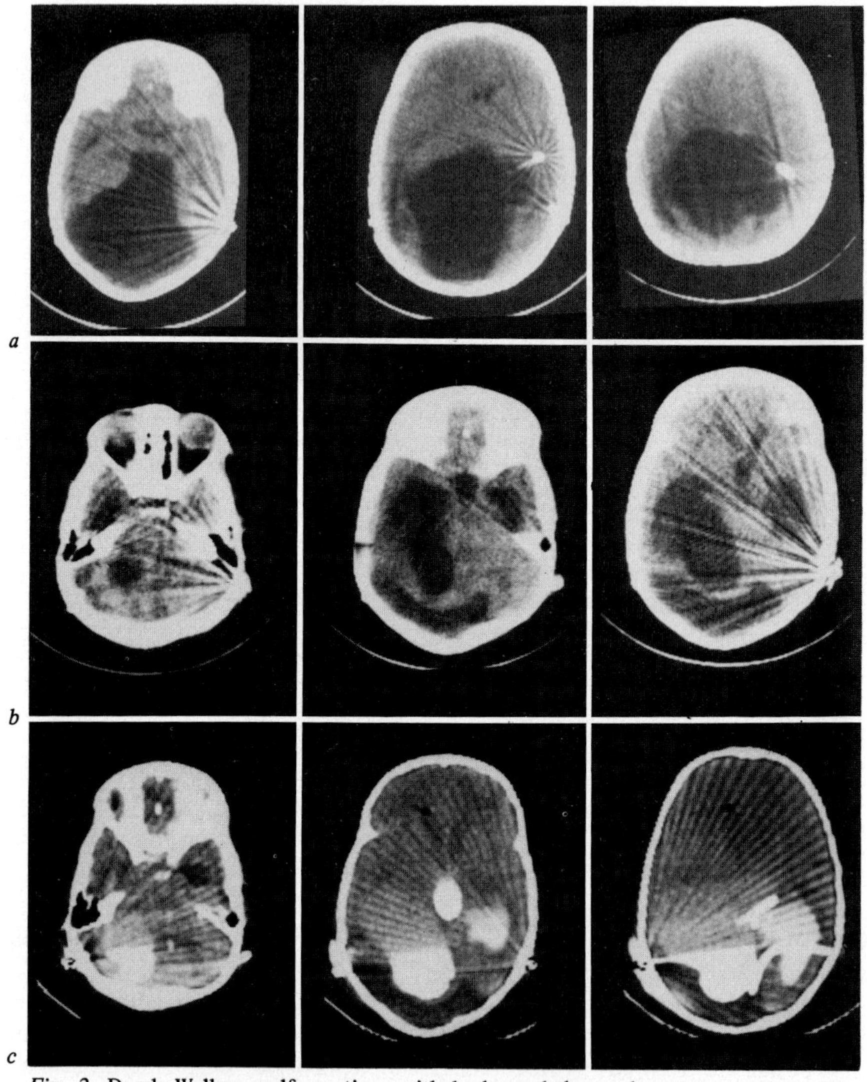

Fig. 2. Dandy-Walker malformation, with hydrocephalus and patent aqueduct. The control scan after drainage of the lateral ventricles shows a tremendous expansion of the Dandy-Walker cyst within the supratentorial cavity (*a*). After shunting, the size of the cyst is markedly reduced, but a low-density area appears in the posterior fossa, while the size of the lateral ventricles is satisfactory (*b*). Opacification of the lateral ventricles with metrizamide shows that this cavity is an expansion of the left lateral ventricle originating from the left choroidal fissure and reaching, through the tentorial notch, the bottom of the posterior fossa, with signs of compression of the brain stem (*c*). Puncture of the left lateral ventricle revealed a normal ventricular pressure. The child eventually died in spite of shunting of the outpouching.

efficiency of the drainage and the possible adverse effects, repeated scanning is not indicated unless EEG or clinical warning signs appear. However, we do not know yet everything about the long-term evolution of these patients and we still have to build our experience about the status of these patients in adulthood.

To conclude, it should be stressed that even after adequate drainage, hydrocephalus is still a possibly evolutive disease. We should like to illustrate this fact by the case of a child who presented with a Dandy-Walker malformation without obstruction of the aqueduct (fig. 2). A ventricular shunting allowed a good resolution of the supratentorial hydrocephalus, but the Dandy-Walker cyst expanded tremendously through the tentorium, between the cerebral hemisphere. A complementary drainage was placed in the posterior fossa, which temporarily relieved the symptoms. But soon the child was admitted again with symptoms related to the brain stem. CT scanning then revealed an outpouching of the tela choroidea of the left lateral ventricle which, through the tentorial notch, occupied most of the posterior fossa, in spite of a normal ventricular pressure, and the child eventually died. Another similar evolution was observed in a case of idiopathic aqueductal occlusion, and was diagnosed at autopsy. Such evolutions, confirm the fact that CT scanning is casting a new light on hydrocephalus, and that ventricular drainage may be disappointing.

C. Raybaud, MD, Service de Neuro-Radiologie de Prof. G. Salamon,
Hôpital de la Timone, Rue Saint Pierre, F–13005 Marseille (France)

Monogr. neural Sci., vol. 8, pp. 144–147 (Karger, Basel 1982)

Computerized Tomography and Shunts

Rafael Carrillo, Luis Nombela, Antonio Rodríguez-Salazar
Clínica Puerta de Hierro, Autonomous University School of Medicine, Madrid, Spain

Because of the precise information it provides about the size and the shape of the ventricular system, computerized tomography (CT scan) is the main test to perform in the evaluation of hydrocephalus in children [2–4, 7]. We are reviewing 80 shunted hydrocephalic children in order to determine the value of the CT scan in its follow-up, trying to inquire how helpful the examination will be before deciding if a shunt should or should not be revised.

Materials and Methods

We selected 80 children with communicating or obstructive hydrocephalus treated by means of a ventriculo-atrial or a ventriculoperitoneal shunt, because each of them had at least one CT scan performed after the operation. In 74 of the 80 cases a preoperative study was also available. We estimated the ventricular size on the CT scan section that includes the frontal horn, measuring the relationship between the distance from the midline to the inner table of the skull and the width of the frontal horn. If it was greater than 3 we classified the ventricles as small; if it was between 3 and 2, as medium size, and when it was under 2, as large. We divided the clinical states of the children into three grades. In grade 'A' the patients showed no symptoms; in grade 'B' the patients showed some neurological defects or moderate psychomotor retardation; patients in grade 'C' were severely retarded or suffered from high intracranial pressure.

From the CT scan we also tried to obtain information about morphological changes and the presence of periventricular lucency. We correlated the preoperative clinical grade in each patient with the ventricular size, the presence of radiolucency and morphological changes on the CT scan performed before surgery. At the time the last CT scan was performed after surgery, we again correlated the clinical grade at that moment with the CT scan changes.

Results

Periventricular lucency appeared only in a few instances, the hydrocephalus being active in these cases, but no significance was found when periventricular

Table I. Patients with small ventricles in the last CT scan performed after shunt

Number of cases and pre-shunt evaluation	Last follow-up evaluation (all small)
8, C (large)	2, C 4, B 2, A
21, B (large)	1, C 5, B 15, A
2 (medium)	2, A
11, B (medium)	4, B 7, A
6 without pre-shunt CT, B	1, B 5, A

A–C = Clinical grades (see text). Large, medium and small refer to size of ventricles.

lucency was not present. From the ventricular morphological analysis no information was obtained concerning the grade of shunt functioning.

Measuring the ventricular size in the last postoperative CT scan, 48 patients had small ventricles, 17 had medium size and 15 had large ones. In the first group 12 remained in the same clinical grade as preoperatively, 35 had changed to a better grade and 1 had from 'B' to 'C' grade, in spite of having improved the ventricles from large to small (table I). Of the 17 with medium size ventricles, 6 cases remained in the same preoperative clinical grade and 11 had improved (table II). Of the 15 cases with large ventricles in their last CT scan, 9 remained in the preoperative clinical grade, 2 had changed to a worse grade and 4 had improved from 'C' or 'B' to 'A' (asymptomatic patients) in spite of having large ventricles (table III). In table IV we show the clinical and CT scan correlations at the time the last postoperative CT scan was performed in the group of 80 patients.

Discussion

When we tried to correlate the clinical category of 80 shunted hydrocephalic children with the size of their ventricles in the CT scan, we found that although most of the patients in the best clinical grade had small ventricles, some of them had medium or even large ones. On the other hand, patients not doing well had

Table II. Patients with medium size ventricles in the last CT scan performed after shunt

Number of cases and pre-shunt evaluation	Last follow-up evaluation (all medium)
5, C (large)	1, C 3, B 1, A
6, B (large)	1, B 5, A
2, C (medium)	1, C 1, B
4, B (medium)	3, B 1, A

A–C = Clinical grades. Large and medium refer to size of ventricles.

Table III. Patients with large ventricles in the last CT scan performed after shunt

Number of cases and pre-shunt evaluation	Last follow-up evaluation (all large)
4, C (large)	3, C 1, A
10, B (large	2, C 5, B 3, A
1, C (medium)	1, C

A–C = Clinical grades. Large and medium refer to size of ventricles.

Table IV. Clinical grade and ventricular size in the last CT scan performed

Ventricle size	Clinical grade			Total
	A	B	C	
Small	32	13	3	48
Medium	7	8	2	17
Large	4	5	6	15
Total	43	26	11	80

large, medium or small size ventricles. Hydrocephalus is the consequence of an increased pressure gradient between the ventricles and the brain [5, 6] and its treatment should diminish or suppress this pressure gradient with secondary reduction of the ventricular volume. When a shunt fails to normalize the pressure, independent of the change in volume of the ventricles, it is working improperly. In a previous paper one of us stressed the importance of diagnosing intraventricular pressure in the follow-up of shunted hydrocephalus [1].

Conclusion

The information provided by a single CT scan, in the absence of periventricular lucency, is insufficient to diagnose an improper functioning of the shunt. It may be necessary to compare carefully repeated studies together with the clinical condition of the patient for evaluating the shunt. Further studies are in progress in order to obtain more benefit from CT scanning in shunted hydrocephalus.

References

1 Carrillo, R.: Cerebral angiography and evaluation of functional status of shunts in hydrocephalic children. Child's Brain *3:* 238–248 (1977).

2 Epstein, F.; Naidich, T.P.; Chase, N.E., et al.: The role of computerized axial tomography in the diagnosis and treatment of common neurosurgical problems in infancy and childhood. Child's Brain *2:* 111–131 (1976).

3 Epstein, F.; Naidich, T.; Kricheff, I., et al.: Role of computerized axial tomography in diagnosis, treatment and follow-up of hydrocephalus. Preliminary communication. Child's Brain *3:* 91–100 (1977).

4 Houser, O.W.; Smith, J.B.; Gomez, H.R. et al.: Evaluation of intracranial disorders in children by computerized transaxial tomography. A preliminary report. Neurology, Minneap. *25:* 607–613 (1975).

5 Milhorat, T.H.: Hydrocephalus and the cerebrospinal fluid, p. 135 (Williams & Wilkins, Baltimore 1972).

6 Raimondi, A.J.: Pediatric neuroradiology, p. 148 (Saunders, Philadelphia 1972).

7 Till, K.: Computerized axial tomography. Particular applications and advantages in pediatric neurosurgery. Child's Brain *2:* 46–53 (1976).

R. Carrillo, MD. Clínica Puerta de Hierro, Autonomous University School of Medicine, Madrid (Spain)

Monogr. neural Sci., vol. 8, pp. 148–152 (Karger, Basel 1982)

Periventricular Lucency in Computed Tomography of Hydrocephalus and Cerebral Atrophy

Koreaki Mori [1], *Hajime Handa* [2], *Takaho Murata* [1], *Yoshihisa Nakano* [3]

[1] Department of Neurosurgery, Kochi Medical School, Kochi
and Department of [2] Neurosurgery and [3] Radiology, Kyoto University, Kyoto, Japan

Introduction

Recently, we recognized that periventricular lucency [2] is encountered not only in hydrocephalus, but also in diseases other than hydrocephalus. Therefore, further observations were made in order to clarify the pathogenesis of periventricular lucency.

Materials and Methods

In 5,470 cases examined by the EMI 1010 head scanner, 191 cases with an enlarged ventricle and 10 cases without ventricular enlargement showed periventricular lucency. Most of the cases without ventricular enlargement were neonatal or infantile epilepsy. In 191 cases with an enlarged ventricle, 62 were cases of hypertensive ventricular dilatation, while the remaining 129 were of the non-hypertensive type. Most of the cases other than hydrocephalus were normal pressure hydrocephalus following subarachnoid hemorrhage and cerebral atrophy. In cases with periventricular lucency, linear density profiles were investigated [1].

Results

In many cases of hypertensive hydrocephalus, there was a decrease in CT number within the periventricular white matter and the component of the ventricular wall could not be identified. Figure 1 shows a linear density profile in the pineal germinoma. In the acute stage of primary and secondary hydrocephalus, periventricular lucency showed a steep rise from the ventricular wall up to the cortical gray matter. After the shunting operation, the inclination of periventricular lucency in the linear density profile became gentle together with a reduction in the size of the ventricles. In chronic hydrocephalus, periventricular lucency

1
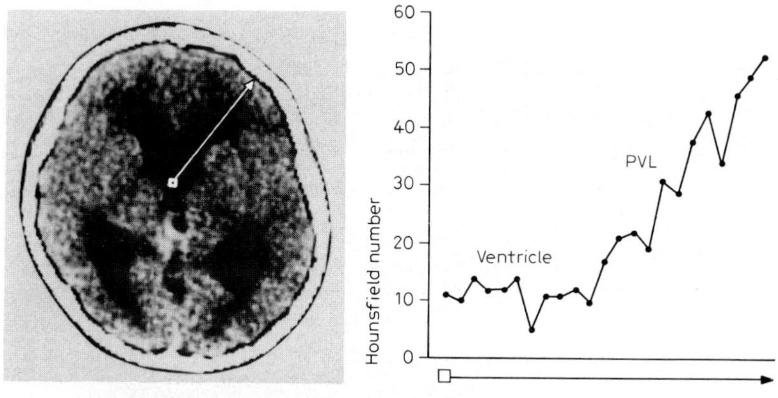

2
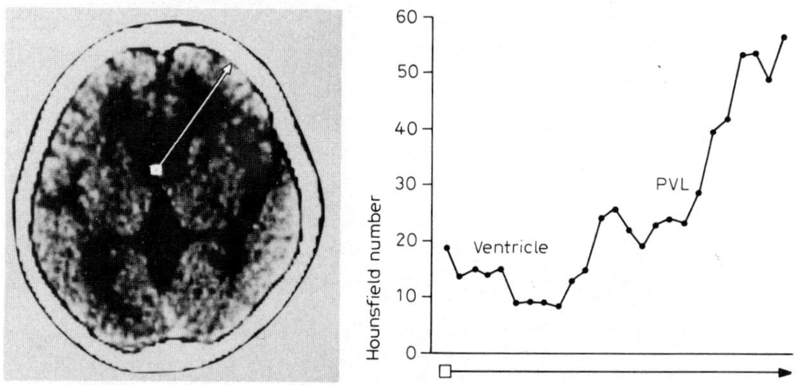

Fig. 1. Pineal germinoma. CT scan (left) shows ventricular dilatation and periventricular lucency of moderate degree. Profile (right) from the ventricle to cortex shows a linear, steep slope.

Fig. 2. Cerebral atrophy. CT scan (left) shows moderate ventricular dilatation and periventricular lucency. Linear density profile (right) from ventricle to cortex shows ventricular wall, followed by periventricular lucency.

was minimal. The inclination of periventricular lucency in chronic hydrocephalus was not so steep as in the acute stage. In normal pressure hydrocephalus, the inclination of periventricular lucency in the linear density profile was gentle as in chronic hydrocephalus.

In the linear density profile of cerebral atrophy, a component corresponding to the ventricular wall was usually noted and the density within the periventricular white matter was flat (fig. 2). In a few cases of cerebral atrophy secondary to hydrocephalus, a gentle inclination was observed as in normal pressure hydrocephalus and the ventricular wall component could not be identified.

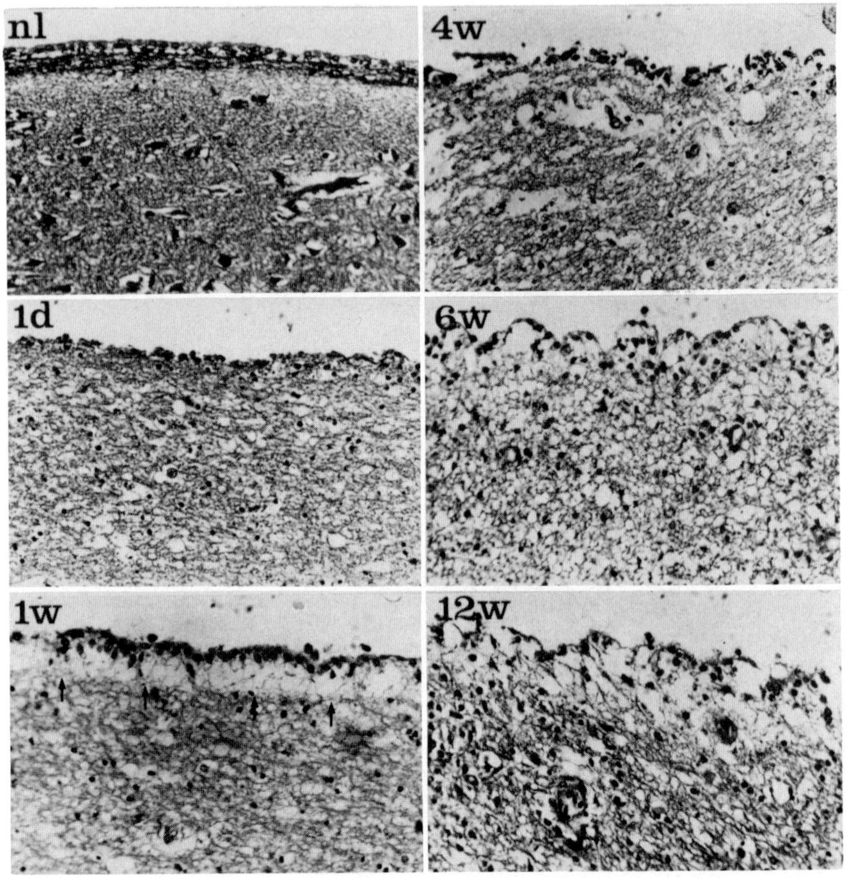

Fig. 3. Light microscopic photographs of superolateral angle of periventricular white matter in various stages of kaolin-induced canine hydrocephalus (normal, 1 day, and 1, 4, 6, and 12 weeks). Arrows indicate spongy and edematous changes in the subependymal layer.

In cases with periventricular lucency without ventricular dilatation, which is often seen in neonatal or young infantile epilepsy, the linear density profile showed a relatively normal parenchymal density between the ventricle and periventricular lucency.

Discussion

Light microscopic examinations of periventricular white matter in canine acute hydrocephalus reveal spongy and edematous changes in the subependymal structures (fig. 3). These changes appear to be consistent with periventricular

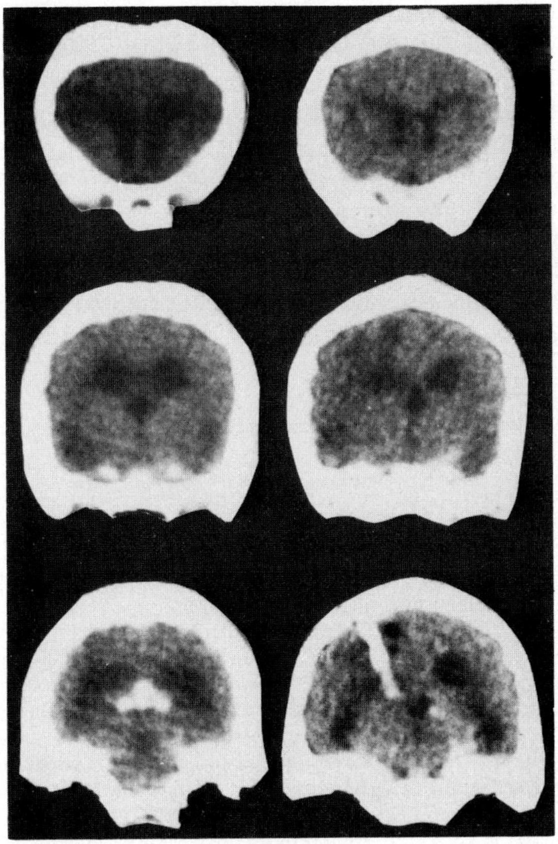

Fig. 4. Observations before (left) and after (right) shunting operation using CT scans. Periventricular lucency immediately disappeared within the second day after operation, accompanied by reduced ventricular size.

lucency in hydrocephalus [5]. Figure 4 shows CT examinations before and after a shunting operation in canine hydrocephalus. Periventricular lucency immediately disappeared within 2–3 days after the operation [4]. Periventricular lucency is a reversible phenomenon and may be regarded as a sign of present or preceding intraventricular hypertension. Periventricular lucency may be a useful finding on CT for the determination of an indication for shunting operation [3].

In some cases of normal pressure hydrocephalus, periventricular lucency was still observed after a reduction of the ventricles. This may represent a parenchymal damage in the white matter rather than water retention and eventual disappearance of periventricular lucency may be caused by reconstruction of the parenchyma.

From the results, periventricular lucency in primary cerebral atrophy may be produced by destructive changes in the white matter, while periventricular lucency in secondary cerebral atrophy may be caused by water retention together with destructive changes in the periventricular white matter. Most cases of cerebral atrophy with periventricular lucency were encountered in aged individuals. This may be explained by the fact that, in older patients, the white matter around the anterior horn may be more vulnerable.

On rare occasions, periventricular lucency is noted also in cases without ventricular dilatation such as neonatal or infantile cases of seizure disorder. This is considered to be hypoxic-ischemic encephalopathy and its pathogenesis relates, in considerable part, to a disturbance in perfusion of the white matter in the arterial borderzone.

References

1 DiChiro, G.; Arimitsu, T.; Brooks, R.A.; Morgenthaler, D.G.; Johnston, A.E.; Keller, M.R.: Computed tomography profiles of periventricular hypodensity in hydrocephalus and leukoencephalopathy. Radiology *130:* 661–666 (1979).

2 Mori, K.; Murata, T.; Handa, H.; Nakano, Y.: Periventricular lucency in hydrocephalus on computerized tomography. Surg. Neurol. *8:* 337–340 (1977).

3 Mori, K.; Handa, H.; Murata, T.; Nakano, Y.: Periventricular lucency in computed tomography of hydrocephalus and cerebral atrophy. J. Comput. assist. Tomogr. *4:* 204–209 (1980).

4 Murata, T.; Mori, K.; Handa, H.; Nakano, Y.: Computed tomography in experimental canine hydrocephalus. 2. Correlation between ventricular enlargement, periventricular lucency and intracranial pressure. Brain Nerve *31:* 313–321 (1979).

5 Murata, T.; Mori, K.; Handa, H.; Nakano, Y.: Computed tomography in experimental canine hydrocephalus. 3. Pathogenesis of periventricular lucency (PVL). Brain Nerve *31:* 721–729 (1979).

K. Mori, MD, Department of Neurosurgery, Kochi Medical School,
Kohasu Okoh-cho Nankoku-City, Kochi 781–51 (Japan)

Monogr. neural Sci., vol. 8. pp. 153–157 (Karger, Basel 1982)

Value of Computed Tomography in Non-Tumorous Hydrocephalus Treated by Ventricular Shunt

B.E. Kendall, D.P.E. Kingsley

Hospital for Sick Children, Great Ormond Street and the London Hospital, Whitechapel, London, England

During the past 5 years computed tomography (CT) has been used to examine 365 children following a ventricular shunt for hydrocephalus, due to a variety of non-tumorous conditions. 182 of these patients had been examined preoperatively and in many cases a number of subsequent CT scans had been performed during the follow-up period. This study was undertaken mainly to determine the limits of satisfactory resolution of CT changes in the uncomplicated cases. Unfortunately, the material in general was unsuitable since limitation on scanning time did not allow routine serial CT and many of the scans were only made when complications were suspected. In a number of these cases an alternative explanation, unrelated to the hydrocephalus or its treatment, was shown to account for the clinical deterioration and together with routine scans in well patients, this group forms the basis of our observations of the satisfactory post shunt course.

Following a ventricular shunt several interacting factors determine the changes in the size of the ventricles. These include: (1) the residual pressure in the ventricle which is related to the resistance in the drainage system, especially the valve; (2) infection which may lead on to ventriculitis and cause loculation with subsequent incomplete ventricular drainage; (3) co-existing brain damage, and (4) extracerebral effusions.

Since the patients have not been scanned at very short intervals our observations are conservative, but it is evident that the rapidity and degree of response of the ventricles to shunting has varied widely. In some children they showed a marked reduction in size within days of insertion of a shunt catheter, the Evans index falling by about 35% within 4 days in 8% of the cases.

Maximum reduction in ventricular size also may occur within a few days; thus 1 patient decreased the Evans index by 30% to a stable value of 0.28; on the other hand, with apparently good shunt function reduction in ventricular size can occur more slowly over a period of weeks, for example a gradual reduc-

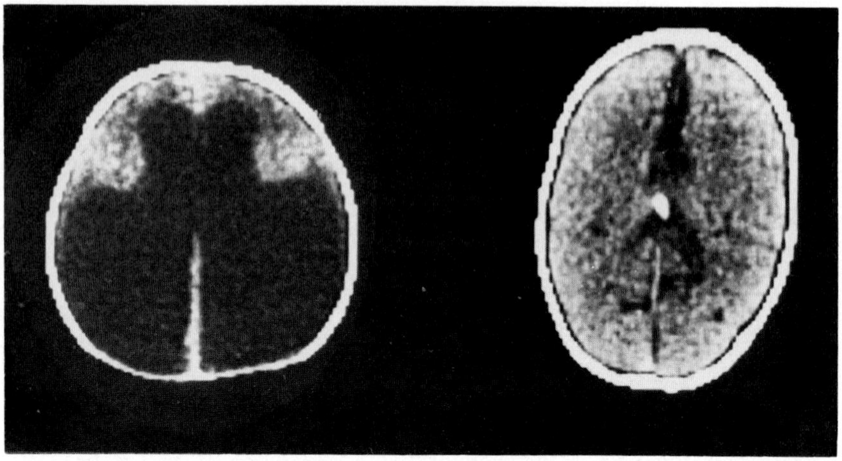

Fig. 1. *a* Infant aged 5 months. Plain CT scan shows gross hydrocephalus particularly involving the trigones and occipital horns. *b* Same patient 1 year later after satisfactory ventriculo-atrial shunt. The ventricles are now of normal size and there is prominence of the interhemispheric fissure anteriorly. The amount of cerebral substance is now normal.

tion of 54% to an Evans index of 0.23 over a 3-week period, or months; thus, in 1 child the minimum size was eventually attained after 5 months.

In several children the hydrocephalus remained unchanged for over a year despite apparently adequate shunts. In some of these the ventricles then became a little smaller without shunt revision. In the others the ventricles remained virtually unchanged over a period of several years with an Evans ratio between 0.35 and 0.5. Shunt revision was not performed because the children were asymptomatic with apparent normal development and the hydrocephalus was considered to have arrested.

The degree of hydrocephalus, as shown on the initial scan, is no guide to the amount of response possible. Even in patients with gross hydrocephalus and as little as 1 mm of thickness of cerebral substance a satisfactory shunt has resulted in a normal ventricular size and cerebral mantle thickness (fig. 1) [2, 10]. In this series the amount of improvement was not age-dependent nor was it related to the cause of the hydrocephalus. Conversely, when raised pressure persisted after a shunt procedure in only 1 case was there an increase in thickness of the cerebral mantle and in another a reduction in size of the ventricles and in both changes were slight (fig. 2, 3). In this particular series there were no patients with a recrudescence of clinically raised intracranial pressure after satisfactory shunting in whom the ventricles remained small [1]. Periventricular lucency was present initially in 28%. Its persistence generally indicated inadequate ventricular drainage [9, 10]. There were two exceptions, one associated with ependymitis, due to

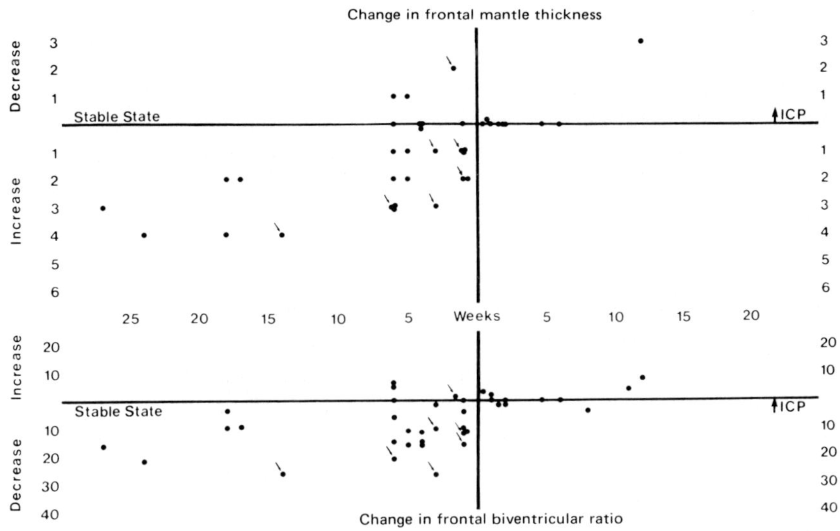

2

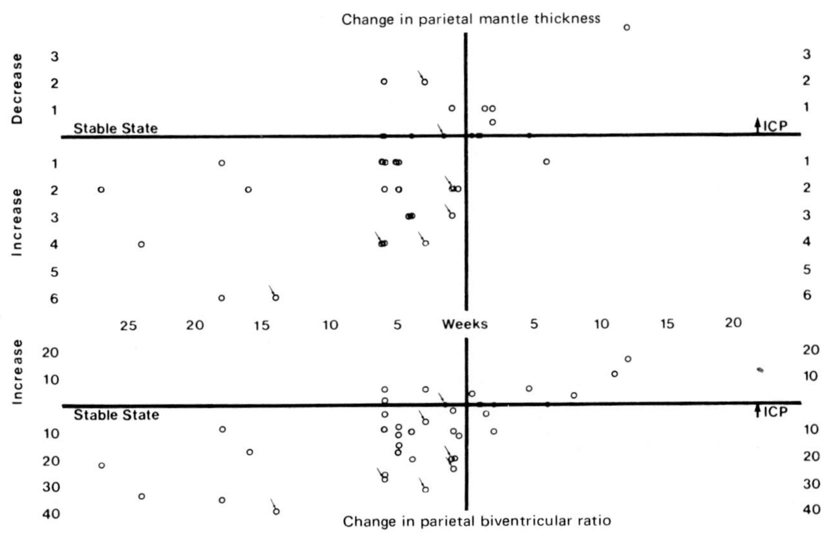

3

Fig. 2, 3. Demonstrating the change in mantle thickness and bi-ventricular ratio in the frontal (fig. 2) and parietal (fig. 3) regions. The changes are related both to the interval between scans and the clinical state of the child. Arrows identify those patients with associated subdural collections. The change in mantle thickness is measured in millimetres on the scan and the change in biventricular ratio as a percentage change from the initial scan.

shunt infection and the other following extensive intraventricular bleeding associated with staphylococcal septicaemia.

Subdural haematomas developed in 12% and in two thirds of these the hydrocephalus was associated with an underlying arachnoid cyst. The minimum interval after the shunt procedure was 6 days; this was in a child with signs of raised intracranial pressure, the Evans index having decreased from 0.68 to a very small size which could not be accurately measured. The other children were scanned between 8 days and 4 months after insertion of the shunt for a variety of reasons, but in no case were there signs of raised intracranial pressure. Similar findings occurred in a previous series [8] in which a number of unsuspected subdurals were revealed on routine follow-up. In our cases most of these developing a subdural haematoma had a relatively rapid reduction in ventricular size.

Where possible the children were assessed both clinically and developmentally and we compared the intellect in those whose ventricles responded satisfactorily to shunting with those whose ventricles remained large. When the ventricles become reduced in size normal intellect is to be expected (83%), but conversely where the ventricles remain large about half (47%) are retarded, although superior intellectual development may be achieved despite extreme hydrocephalus [6]. The presence of subdural haematomas did not appear to affect the outcome, but it is generally acknowledged that early shunting does [5, 12].

The underlying cause of the hydrocephalus has a wide pathogenetic basis, but unlike *Mealey et al.* [7] we were unable to show a relationship between the primary pathology and the behaviour of the shunt or the long-term mental development of the child. There was no relation between the number of shunt revisions and the final outcome provided that adequate drainage was achieved.

The shunt became infected in 24% of cases; only 25% of these had a satisfactory reduction in ventricular size and half were retarded; 75% showed no response and of these only a third developed normally, the others either died or were retarded, confirming the poorer outlook previously recorded [3, 11].

This limited study demonstrates that shunt procedures should be repeated as necessary to produce satisfactory drainage of hydrocephalus and that there is no evidence that multiple procedures detract from the final outcome [4]. Provided significant brain damage has not already occurred many of these children can develop normally; close and repeated CT evaluation should be undertaken until arrest is documented.

References

1 Epstein, F.J.; Fleischer, A.S.; Hochwald, G.M.; Ransohoff, J.: Subtemporal craniectomy for recurrent shunt obstruction secondary to small ventricles. J. Neurosurg. *41:* 29–31 (1974).

2 Epstein, F.J.; Rubin, R.C.; Hochwald, G.M.: Restoration of cortical mantle in severe feline hydrocephalus; a new laboratory method. Devl Med. Child Neurol. *32:* suppl., pp. 49–53 (1974).
3 Foltz, E.L.; Shurtleff, D.B.: Five year comparative study of hydrocephalus in children with and without operation. J. Neurosurg. *20:* 1064–1078 (1963).
4 Guiffrè, R.; Palma, L.; Fontana, M.: Extracranial CSF shunting for infantile non-tumoural hydrocephalus. A retrospective analysis of 360 cases. Clin. Neurol. Neurosurg. *81:* 199–210 (1979).
5 Lawrence, K.M.: The natural history of hydrocephalus. Lancet *ii:* 1152–1154 (1958).
6 Lorber, J.: The results of early treatment of extreme hydrocephalus. Devl Med. Child Neurol. *16:* suppl., pp. 21–29 (1968).
7 Mealey, J.; Gilmor, R.L.; Bubb, M.P.: The prognosis of hydrocephalus overt at birth. J. Neurosurg. *39:* 348–355 (1973).
8 Moseley, I.F.: The use of computed tomography scanning in the postoperative assessment of patients with ventricular shunts. Extract *3:* 15–21 (1978).
9 Naidich, T.P.; Epstein, F.J.; Lin, J.P.; Kritcheff, I.I.; Hochwald, G.M.: Evaluation of paediatric hydrocephalus by computerised tomography. Radiology *119:* 337–345 (1976).
10 Palmieri, A.; Menichelli, F.; Pasquini, U.; Salvolini, U.: The role of computed tomography in the postoperative evaluation of infantile hydrocephalus. Neuroradiology *14:* 257–262 (1978).
11 Tsingoglu, S.; Forrest, D.A.: Complications from Holter ventriculo-atrial shunts. Br. J. Surg. *58:* 372–377 (1971).
12 Young, H.F.; Nulsen, F.E.; Weiss, M.H.; Thomas, P.: The relationship of intelligence and cerebral mantle in treated infantile hydrocephalus. Paediatrics, Springfield *52:* 38–44 (1974).

B.E. Kendall, MD, Hospital for Sick Children, London Hospital,
Great Ormond Street, Whitechapel, London (England)

Monogr. neural Sci., vol. 8, pp. 158–169 (Karger, Basel 1982)

Technical Problems in Shunts

Harold J. Hoffman

Division of Neurosurgery, Hospital for Sick Children; University of Toronto, Toronto, Canada

Introduction

The commonest cause of cerebrospinal fluid (CSF) by-pass shunt malfunction is improper surgical technique for the initial placement of the shunt. This cause far outnumbers the other etiologies of shunt malfunction and is obviously a preventable cause of shunt malfunction.

Lumboperitoneal Shunts

The use of shunts from lumbar subarachnoid space to the peritoneal cavity was initially described by *Ferguson* [1] in 1898. The fear of arachnoiditis and spinal curvature, however, has dissuaded most individuals from relying on this form of shunting device.

The great advantages of lumboperitoneal shunts are the small area of the body that requires exposure for implantation of the tube and consequently the reduced risk of shunt infection. The initial tubes, however, were made of polyethylene which is a notoriously irritating material, and led to a very significant rate of arachnoiditis resulting in neurological deficit and spinal curvature [2]. Furthermore, these initial polyethylene shunts were valveless which frequently led to low-pressure states intracranially with cephalocranial disproportion as well as shunt dependency [3].

Since 1973, we have been implanting a T-shaped lumboperitoneal shunt by laminectomy [4]. We initially placed the T end of the shunt in the upper lumbar region but feel it is more advantageous to place it at the L4–5 level (fig. 1). The tubing is non-kinkable and is 65 cm long so that an adequate length can be left in the peritoneal cavity. The T in the subarachnoid space prevents migration of the tube, a problem found with the percutaneously placed lumboperitoneal

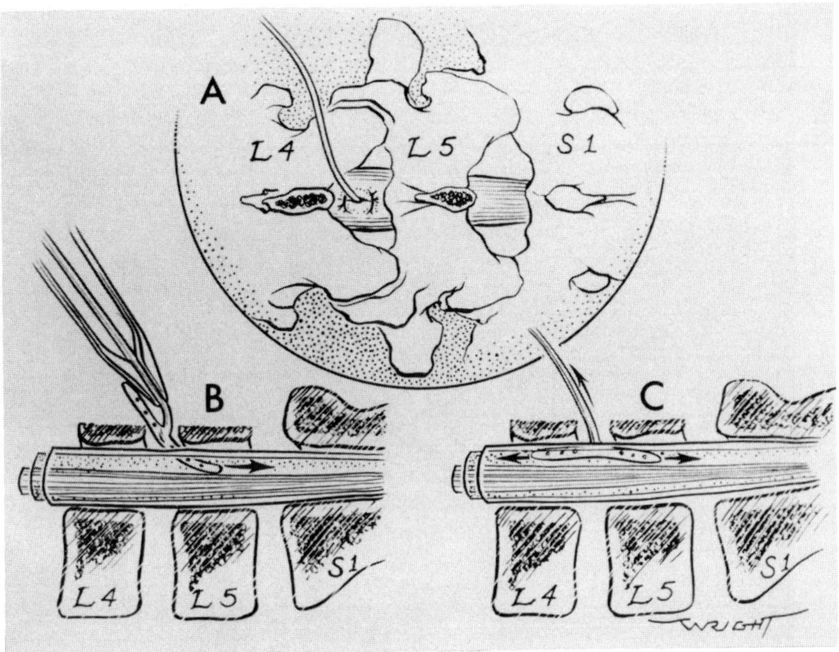

Fig. 1. Technique of placement of lumbar end of T-tube. LP shunt: *A* site of laminectomy; *B, C* method of introduction of lumbar end of shunt.

shunts [5]. A T-shaped lumboperitoneal shunt placed in an infant can typically function for many years without risk of migration or obstruction due to growth.

In the older child with communicating hydrocephalus and large ventricles, a valved T-tube will still occasionally produce a low-pressure state. This can now be corrected with the Cordis (Cordis Corporation, Miami, Fla.) high-low pressure device which is incorporated in the T-tube and changes the pressure dynamics when the patient is upright or recumbent.

Ventricular Shunt

Shunts from the lateral ventricles are typically led either into the peritoneal cavity or into the right atrium of the heart. For proper function of these ventricular cathethers, they must be well placed. In the young infant with enormous ventricles, one can theoretically place the catheter through a burr hole at any site in the head and get a good brisk flow of CSF. However, with the passage of time, the cerebral mantle is reconstituted and if the ventricular catheter is not properly placed, ideally in the frontal horn, it will block. This is the commonest cause of shunt obstruction in my experience.

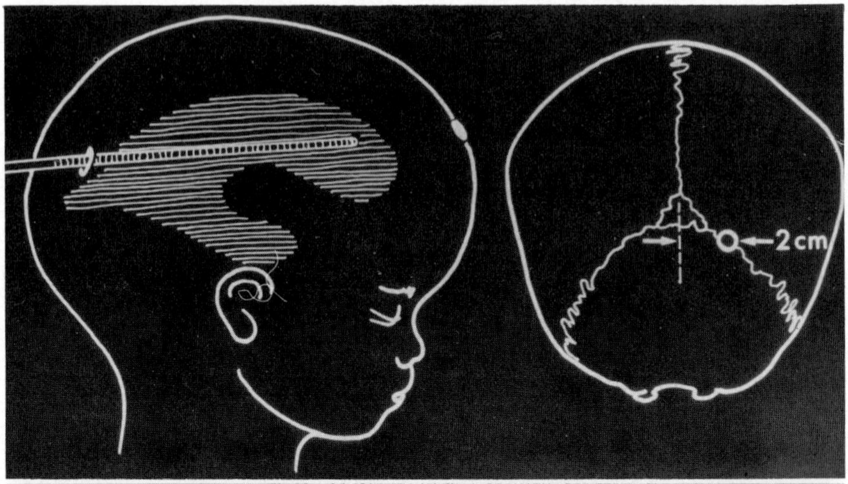

2

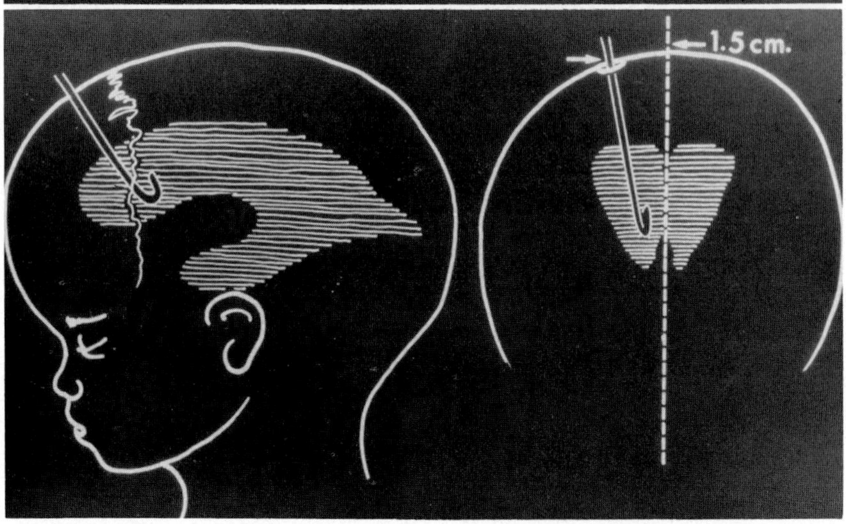

3

Fig. 2. **Technique of introducing ventricular catheter from occipital region into frontal horn.**

Fig. 3. Technique of introducing ventricular catheter from frontal region into frontal horn.

In the young infant with large ventricles, we usually introduce the ventricular catheter into the frontal horn through a small opening in the lambdoid suture (fig. 2). It is essential that this opening be some 2 cm from the midline and that the trajectory of the catheter be towards the midline of the forehead, half way between nasion and hairline. Such a trajectory will carry the catheter into the frontal horn providing the catheter has been measured to reach just beyond the foramen of Monro, typically at the level of the coronal suture.

In order for the trajectory to be maintained, a stylet must be in the catheter until the final target is reached. Slipping the catheter in freehand will lead to a high incidence of shunts located in the temporal horn. We have even had one shunt led into a suprapineal recess which was then threaded down the aqueduct inadvertently so that the tip of the catheter lodged in the fourth ventricle.

In older children, particularly when the ventricles are small, we feel that it is unwise to pass a catheter from occipital bone through to the frontal horn. For this reason, we prefer a frontal burr hole some 1.5 cm from the midline, just behind the hairline and well in front of coronal suture (fig. 3). From this burr hole, the catheter is directed medially and somewhat posteriorly into frontal horn. The ideal catheter for such a frontal horn trajectory is the Hakim (Cordis Corporation, Miami, Fla.) shepherd's crook cathether which will assume the shepherd's crook shape once the stylet is removed and thus prevent the catheter from breaking through ependyma, or going through the foramen of Monro. We have had catheters placed in the third ventricle inadvertently which have failed to deal adequately with the patient's hydrocephalus, and we therefore feel that the catheters must be placed in frontal horn.

In the past, we frequently used the connector at skull level connecting this either with a right angle connector to a flat pump, or with a straight connector to a pump in the burr hole. The disadvantage of such connections is that with revisions, ventricular cathethers frequently became lost. This was of particular nuisance if the shunt was infected and the lost catheter had to be recovered, either by craniotomy or with the aid of a ventriculoscope.

We now do not use a connector at skull level, but rather lead the ventricular catheter out of the burr hole onto the skull surface and connect it by means of a straight connector onto a flat pump.

Slit Ventricle

Shunts led from the ventricle, no matter what their pressure, will lead to a siphoning effect with the production of a negative intracranial pressure and the development of slit-like ventricles in time (fig. 4). The use of an antisiphon will tend to prevent this problem (fig. 5). However, antisiphon devices cannot be used in the young infant, where in fact a negative pressure is desirable to help reconstitute the cerebral mantle. In the older child, however, with large ventricles and a fixed calvarium, the antisiphon device becomes mandatory to prevent low-pressure states resulting in slit ventricles and also to prevent subdural hematomas which occur in these low-pressure states. Shunts into the peritoneal cavity extend a longer distance from the cranial cavity than shunts into the atrium, and thus have a much higher incidence of siphoning problems.

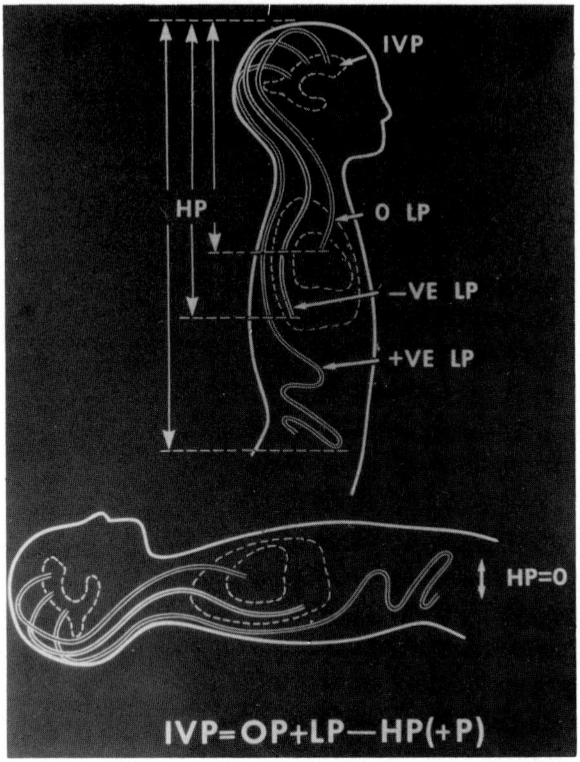

Fig. 4. Diagrammatic explanation of siphoning effect. IVP = intraventricular pressure; HP = hydrostatic pressure; P = atmospheric pressure; LP = pressure in lumen into which shunt is led; atrial pressure = O, pleural pressure = negative, peritoneal pressure = positive; OP = opening pressure in valve of shunting device.

Shunt Infection

Shunt infection is due to a combination of factors. These include the area of body surface which must be prepared and draped for insertion of the shunt, the length of time needed to insert the shunt, and the amount of surgical trauma that is necessary for insertion of the shunt.

Lumboperitoneal shunts, having very small areas of skin to be prepared and draped, are less prone to shunt infections than VP shunts or VA shunts. The exposed skin must be adequately washed. On our service, the children are bathed with phisohex several times before they are brought to the operating room for a

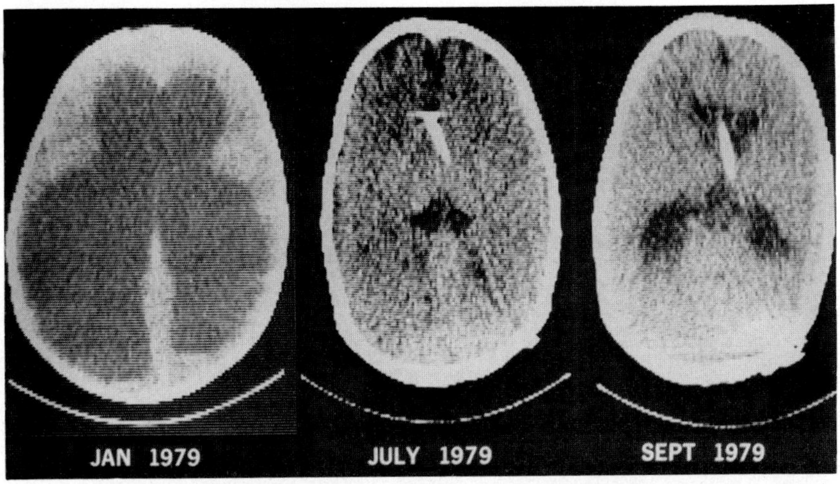

Fig. 5. Dramatic change in ventricular size from January 1979 to July 1979 after insertion of VP shunt. Following insertion of antisiphon device ventricles show mild enlargement (September, 1979).

shunt procedure. At the time of surgery, a fat solvent is used to remove grease and debris from the skin in the operative field. Following adequate washing and draping of the exposed area, an adhesive sterile plastic drape is applied to the skin to keep it out of the operative field. It is essential to use as few incisions as possible in order to avoid contamination of tubing with skin organisms. We use a long shunt passer which can pass a shunt from the cranial cavity to the abdomen without any interposing incisions, even in an adult (fig. 6).

The use of prophylactic antibiotics remains controversial even though our retrospective study indicates that their use reduces shunt infections. A prospective double-blind study will clearly be necessary to solve the dilemma about the use of prophylactic antibiotics. However, I think that all would agree that the implanted tubing must be sterile. For this reason, the tubing during surgery should be kept in a bath of antibiotic solution which is adequately covered and protected from organisms that might be in the operating room air.

Ventriculoperitoneal Shunts

The peritoneal cavity occasionally will not absorb CSF, leading to ascites. The usual cause that we have found for this problem has been a protein secreting tumor, typically an optic nerve glioma.

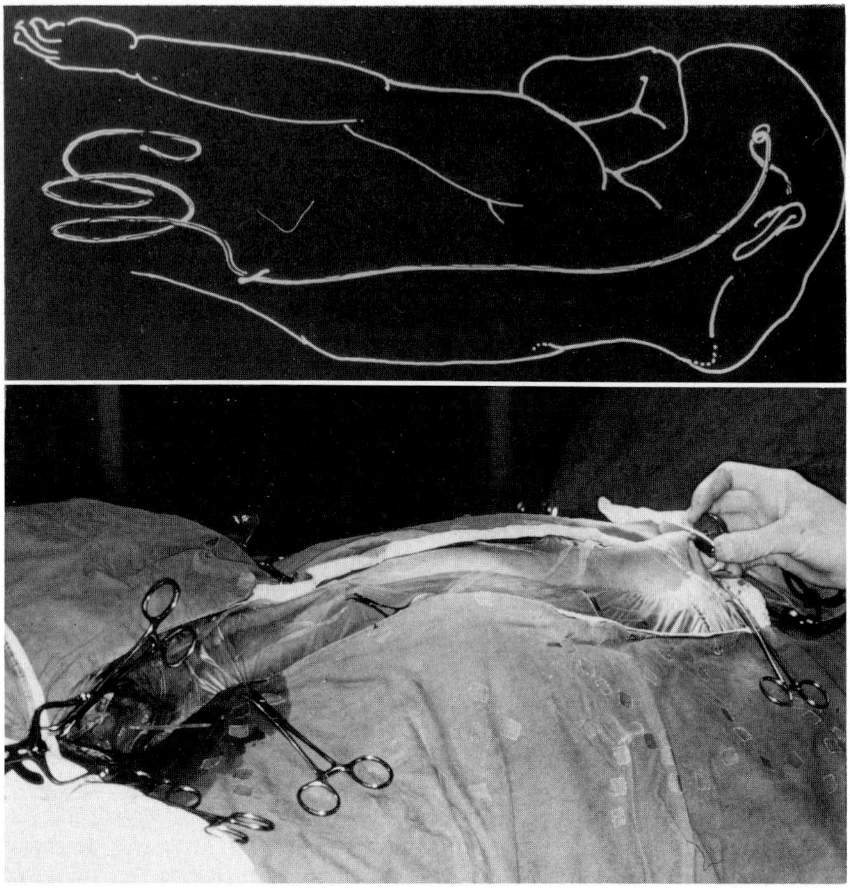

a

b

Fig. 6. a Diagrammatic demonstration of technique for passing VP shunt. *b* Operative photograph showing shunt passer in place.

Catheters in the peritoneal cavity can erode into various viscera. Our experience includes erosion through bowel and protrusion out through anus (fig. 7), into stomach from whence they are vomited through the mouth, and penetration through umbilicus. If there is a previous predisposition to herniation through the inguinal canal, the influx of CSF into the peritoneal cavity will certainly contribute to the development of a hernia. Shunts can lead tumor cells into the peritoneal cavity, but a millipore filter will prevent this complication in susceptible patients [6].

The development of a one-piece shunt has led to diminished breakage of tubing and disconnection at connectors. The original one-piece ventriculo-

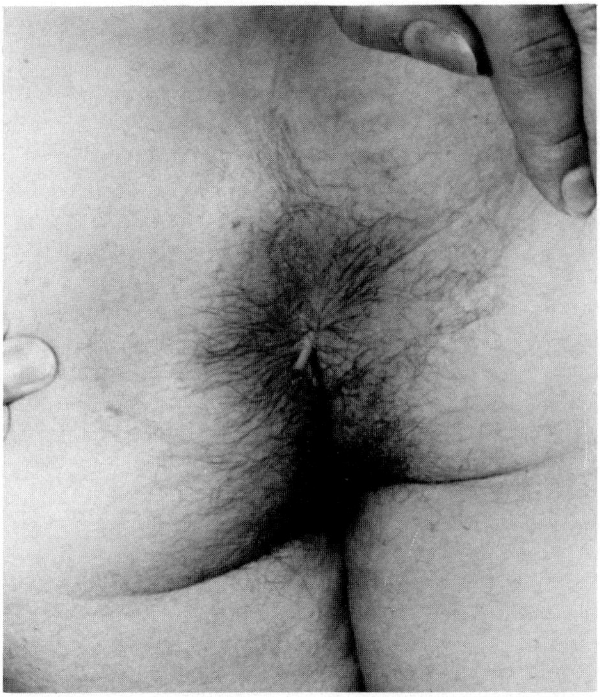

Fig. 7. Peritoneal catheter protruding through anus and still draining CSF.

peritoneal shunt had no reservoir, preventing studies such as shunt scans and percutaneous testing of shunt function. Furthermore, it is occasionally necessary to inject antibiotics into a shunt and this was not available in the one-piece shunt without a reservoir.

We have been implanting a one-piece shunt with a reservoir (Codman & Shurtleff, Inc., Randolph, Mass.) which allows for clinical testing of the shunting device as well as retrieval of CSF and injection of agents for diagnostic studies. The one-piece shunt should avoid the problems of disconnection and breakage (fig. 8).

The use of a trochar for introduction of the peritoneal catheter exposes the patient to the risk of bowel perforation and the resultant morbidity and mortality of shunt infection. At our institution, all peritoneal catheters are introduced by direct operative exposure which can be done easily and quickly in the infant and child. With this technique, we have never encountered operative perforation of bowel.

a

b

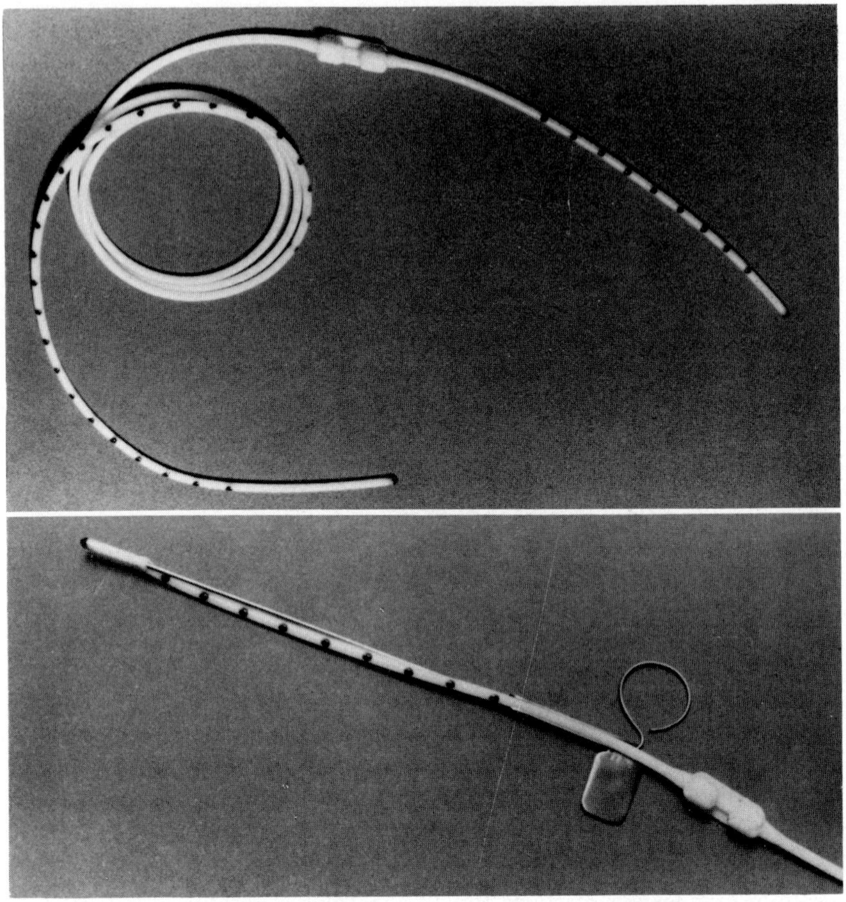

Fig. 8. a New one-piece shunt with reservoir. *b* Special stylet for introducing ventricular end of one-piece shunt into frontal horn.

Ventriculo-Atrial Shunts

Ventriculo-atrial shunts are much less prone to the siphoning effect that plagues the ventriculoperitoneal shunt. However, if the valve of the ventriculo-atrial shunt becomes incompetent, blood can reflux up the tube and clog the shunt. If such a clogged shunt is pumped, clots can be extruded into the lungs producing pulmonary emboli. If a ventriculo-atrial shunt gets infected, infected pulmonary emboli occur leading to pulmonary infarcts (fig. 9). Eventually, mul-

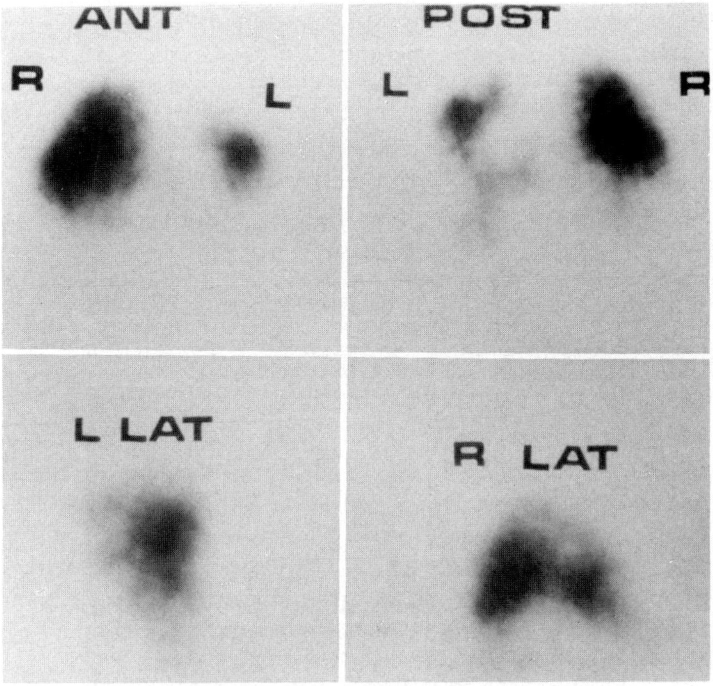

Fig. 9. Lung scan demonstrating multiple pulmonary infarcts in child with VA shunt.

tiple pulmonary infarcts result in pulmonary hypertension and cor pulmonale. With an infected ventriculo-atrial shunt, emboli can occur eventually in various body viscera leading to petechial hemorrhages in skin, and shunt nephritis.

Third Ventriculoscopy

Because of the many problems that the child with shunt dependency and non-communicating hydrocephalus is prone to, we have advocated percutaneous third ventriculostomy for those children with non-communicating hydrocephalus who have a large third ventricle that lends itself to a percutaneous third ventriculostomy [7]. The advantage of this technique is that it is safe and effective in the majority of patients with non-communicating hydrocephalus who have a large third ventricle which herniates down over the dorsum sellae. Since the procedure is carried out stereotactically, we have found that there is little in the way of risk to brain parenchyma during the procedure (fig. 10).

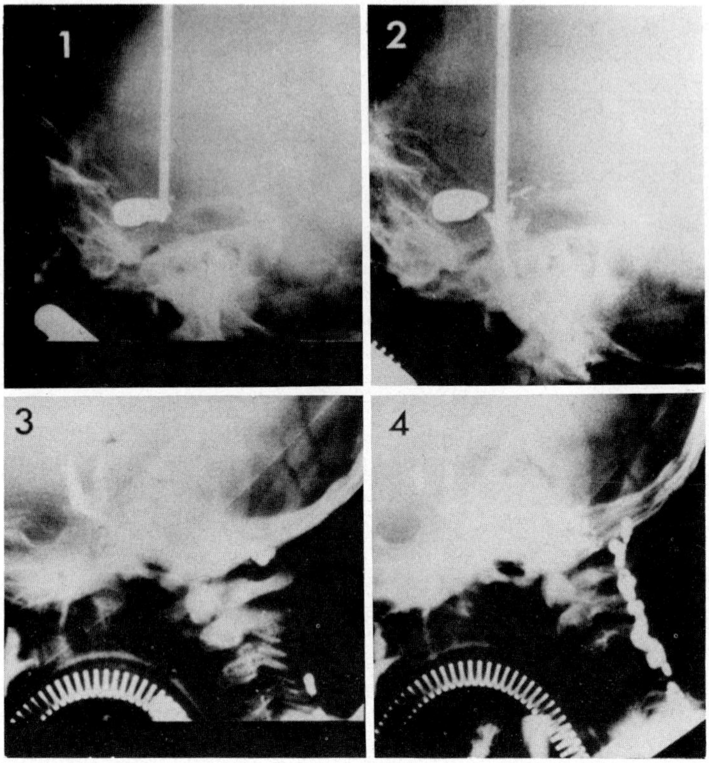

Fig. 10. Operative steps in percutaneous third ventriculostomy. *1* Leukotome resting on floor of third ventricle which is filled with pantopaque. *2* Floor of third ventricle has been punctured and pantopaque has flowed into basal cisterns. *3, 4* After removal of leukotome, pantopaque flows from third ventricle out into basal cisterns and spinal subarachnoid space.

Conclusion

The management of hydrocephalus is dependent not only on the variety of shunting devices that we use, but on the technical skill of the surgeon inserting the device. With the growth of pediatric neurosurgery, the technical skills for proper insertion of a shunting device will no doubt become universally available. Even then, however, we will be faced with the problems created by mechanical malfunction of shunts. In time, the ideal shunting device will be found which will be free of mechanical problems, and if placed in a technically satisfactory fashion, will be free of many of the problems that our present shunting systems provide.

References

1 Ferguson, A.H.: Intraperitoneal diversion of cerebrospinal fluid in cases of hydrocephalus. N.Y. Med. J. *67:* 902 (1908).
2 Kushner, J.; Alexander, E., Jr., Davis, C.H., Jr.; Kelly, D.L., Jr.: Kyphoscoliosis following lumbar subarachnoid shunts. J. Neurosurg. *34:* 783–791 (1971).
3 Tucker, W.; Hoffman, H.J.: Cephalocranial disproportion. A complication of the treatment of hydrocephalus in children. Child's Brain *2:* 167–176 (1976).
4 Hoffman, H.J.; Hendrick, E.B.; Humphreys, R.P.: New lumboperitoneal shunt for communicating hydrocephalus. J. Neurosurg. *44:* 258–261 (1976).
5 Spetzler, R.F.; Wilson, C.B.; Schulte, R.: Simplified percutaneous lumboperitoneal shunting. Surg. Neurol. *7:* 25–29 (1977).
6 Hoffman, H.J.; Hendrick, E.B.; Humphreys, R.P.: Metastasis via ventriculoperitoneal shunt in patients with medulloblastoma. J. Neurosurg. *44:* 562–566 (1976).
7 Hoffman, H.J.: The advantages of percutaneous third ventriculostomy over other forms of surgical treatment of infantile obstructive hydrocephalus; in Morley, Current controversies in neurosurgery, pp. 691–703 (Saunders, Philadelphia 1976).

H.J. Hoffman, MD, Division of Neurosurgery, Hospital for Sick Children
and University of Toronto, Toronto (Canada)

Monogr. neural Sci., vol. 8, pp. 170–178 (Karger, Basel 1982)

Percutaneous Ventriculocisternostomies in Non-Communicating Hydrocephalus

Jean-François Hirsch

Hôpital Necker Enfants-Malades, Paris, France

Since the work of *Nulsen and Spitz* [23], and the introduction of the Holter valve in 1956, the treatment of hydrocephalus has become more efficient. Indeed most neurosurgeons now consider all other surgical procedures to be obsolete. However, it is also now obvious that the overall mortality and morbidity from ventricular shunting is far from negligible. Therefore, the belief that extracranial shunts represent the only surgical treatment in all cases of hydrocephalus should be reexamined. I will try to show that for some cases of non-communicating hydrocephalus there is an alternative. This is percutaneous third ventriculocisternostomy.

In our opinion extracranial shunts remain the only available procedure in communicating hydrocephalus since the efficiency of choroid plexus cauterization [2, 5, 26, 29] is still not proven. However, this is not true in non-communicating hydrocephalus which can, in some cases, benefit from an intracranial shunt. To decide which should be used, it is then necessary to compare the different procedures, their risks and efficiency, short-term and long-term. In this discussion, it should be kept in mind that even though valves carry a low short-term postoperative mortality, the overall mortality varies from 16 to 20%; over 50% of the children will have to undergo operative intervention several times because of infection, occlusion or other causes of mechanical dysfunction. Moreover, complications such as subdural effusions, secondary craniosynostosis, or slit ventricles are due to inability of extracranial shunts to restore a normal CSF circulation. The problem therefore is to find an intracranial shunt which, in non-communicating hydrocephalus, will be less risky and more efficient. If such a procedure could be found, it would then be necessary to determine when it could be rationally utilized, since it has been claimed that, in congenital aqueductal stenosis, the subarachnoid spaces are not competent and that some cases of non-communicating hydrocephalus are secondary to communicating hydrocephalus [36].

Table I. Direct ventriculocisternostomies with open craniotomy

Author	Year	Ventricle	Cistern
Dandy	1922	3rd →	chiasmatic
Dandy	1932	3rd →	interpeduncular
Stookey and Scarff	1936	3rd →	chiasmatic and interpeduncular
Guillaume	1941	3rd →	chiasmatic
White and Michelsen	1942	3rd →	galenic ambient
Hyndman	1946	lateral →	venae parvae

Intracranial shunts may be divided into three groups: Those which create a direct communication between the ventricular cavities and the subarachnoid spaces, and require an open craniotomy (direct ventriculocisternostomies); those which create a communication via a drain (indirect ventriculocisternostomies); those which create a communication via a drain (indirect ventriculocisternostomies); the direct ventriculocisternostomies, which can be performed under endoscopic or X-ray guidance through a percutaneous approach. Several direct ventriculocisternostomies (table I), with an open craniotomy, have been proposed since *Dandy* [3]. Most of them create a communication between the third ventricle and the chiasmatic or the interpeduncular cistern. However, they failed in one third of the cases and mortality was high (15%). Moreover, the cistern into which the third ventricle was opened was usually destroyed by the surgical approach.

Among the various indirect ventriculostomies (table II) the most widely used has been the Torkildsen procedure. The cases reviewed by *Scarff* [31] indicated that mortality was 25%, mechanical dysfunction 50% and the incidence of failure 40%. It should be noted, however, that this review dates back to 1966. *Lapras et al.* [17] and *Lapras* [18], reviving the Dandy aqueductal catheterization, demonstrated that the postoperative mortality could be lowered to 5%, thus demonstrating that this technique can be useful in special cases. However, it is obvious that most of these techniques entail a high mortality rate and cannot replace, especially in infants, extracranial shunts.

Table II. Indirect ventriculocisternostomies

Author	Year	Ventricle		Ventricle or cistern
Dandy	1918	3rd	→	4th v.
Torkildsen	1939	lateral	→	c. magna
Riechert	1949	lateral	→	c. magna
Leksell	1949	3rd	→	4th v.
Feld	1951	lateral	→	c. chiasmatic
Lazorthes et al.	1957	lateral	→	c. of the corpus callosum
Forjaz et al.	1968	3rd	→	c. interpeduncular
Brocklehurst	1974	lateral	→	c. chiasmatic
Lapras et al.	1975	3rd	→	4th v.

Direct percutaneous ventriculocisternostomies (table III) do not suffer such criticism and might be therefore the alternative in some cases of non-communicating hydrocephalus. This technique was used for the first time by *Mixter* [22] in 1923, with an endoscopic guidance, and by *McNickle* [21] in 1947 under X-ray control. It was revived by *Guiot* [13] and *Guiot et al.* [11, 12] and then used by other neurosurgeons [15]. We started using this technique in 1973, and our experience is now based upon 90 ventriculocisternostomies with a follow-up of 7 years for the first patients. As do most authors, we create a communication between the third ventricle and the interpeduncular cistern with a leukotome thrust through the floor of the third ventricle (fig. 1). Some authors [27, 37], however, open the lamina terminalis, a procedure that we would not recommend because it is less efficient and more hazardous.

The main argument favoring percutaneous ventriculostomies is its low mortality. Reviewing the 236 cases of percutaneous ventriculocisternostomies published (table IV) we calculated an overall mortality rate of 1.3%. This rate can be lowered if the patients are well selected. The technique should only be performed when the third ventricle is large and when its floor bulges into the interpeduncular cistern. Then the hypothalamic nervous structures are displaced laterally; the floor on the midline consists only of pia mater and the puncture can be undertaken without risk [13]. In our 45 last ventriculocisternostomies, thus selected, the mortality was nil. It should also be stressed that the long-term mortality is low. The 4.4% overall mortality rate in our series of ventriculo-

Table III. Direct ventriculocisternostomies without open craniotomy

Author	Year	Guidance	Perforation
Mixter	1923	endoscopic	floor of 3rd ventricle
Scarff	1936	endoscopic	floor of 3rd ventricle
McNickle	1947	X-ray	floor of 3rd ventricle
Guiot et al.	1963	endoscopic	floor of 3rd ventricle
Guiot et al.	1968	X-ray	floor of 3rd ventricle
Hoffman	1974	X-ray	floor of 3rd ventricle
Pierre-Kahn et al.	1975	X-ray	floor of 3rd ventricle
Sayers and Kosnick	1976	X-ray	lamina terminalis and floor of 3rd ventricle
Vries	1978	endoscopic	floor of 3rd ventricle
Ziedses des Plantes and Crezee	1978	X-ray	lamina terminalis

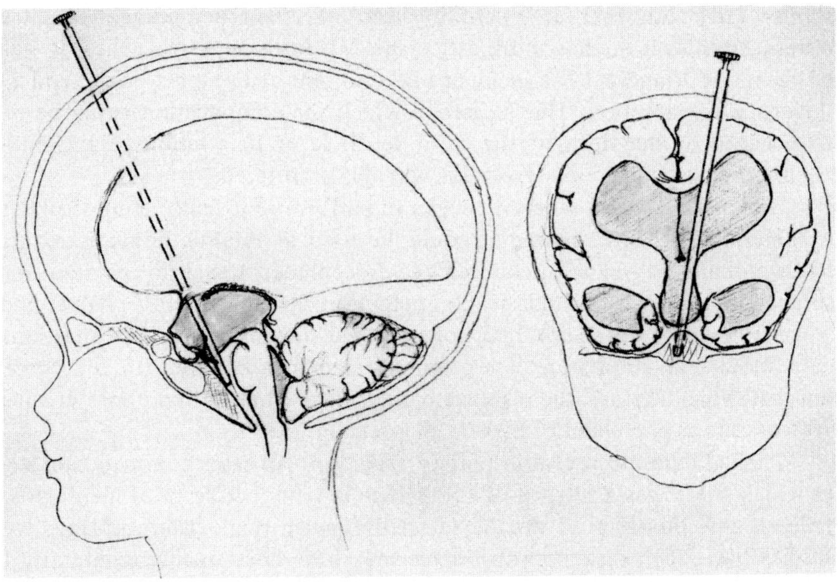

Fig. 1. Communication between the third ventricle and the interpeduncular cistern is achieved by a leukotome thrust through the floor of the third ventricle.

Table IV. Mortality in percutaneous direct ventriculocisternostomy

Author	Year	Number of cases	Mortality	
			number	%
Mixter	1923	1	0	0
Scarff	1936	1	0	0
McNickle	1947	7	0	0
Guiot et al./Guiot	1968/1973	14	0	0
Hoffman	1974	11	0	0
Pierre-Kahn et al./Hirsch et al.	1975/1980	90	2	2.2
Sayers and Kosnik	1976	46	1	2.1
Ziedses des Plantes and Crezee	1978	61	0	0
Vries	1978	5	0	0
Total		236	3	1.3

cisternostomies should be compared to the 16% rate in our series of extracranial shunts [14]. Another argument in favor of direct percutaneous ventriculo-cisternostomies is the low morbidity (table V). Again, reviewing the 236 published cases, we found a 1.7% incidence of transient oculomotor palsies and a 0.8% incidence of infection. The 7 cases in which the complication could be related to a lesion of the floor of the third ventricle or to a lesion of the midbrain occurred when the lamina terminalis was also perforated.

Our main concern when we began to perform ventriculocisternostomies was to determine if this technique could be used in infant's non-communicating hydrocephalus as well as in children's hydrocephalus. It was not obvious that the subarachnoid spaces would be competent in infant's hydrocephalus, and the work of *Guiot et al.* [12] had not provided the answer to that question. Our data show that infants are less often selected than children for the operation, but that, when they are, the results are only slightly better than those in children: 70% success as compared to 80% in children.

Clinical data are useful in patient selection. All cases of aqueductal stenosis in which there was a history of subarachnoid hemorrhage or of meningitis were failures and thus should not be selected for ventriculocisternostomy. Isotope studies have been disappointing, since they have been unable to identify those cases in which the subarachnoid space was collapsed because of an increased intraventricular pressure from those in which it was definitely obstructed.

Table V. Complications in percutaneous direct ventriculocisternostomy

Author	Year	Number of cases	Complication
Mixter	1923	1	0
Scarff	1936	1	0
McNickle	1947	7	0
Guiot et al./Guiot	1968/1973	14	0
Hoffman	1974	11	1 transient 3rd nerve weakness
Pierre-Kahn et al./Hirsch et al.	1975/1980	90	1 transient 3rd nerve weakness 2 meningitis 3 subdural hydroma
Sayers and Kosnick	1976	46	1 transient inappropriate ADH response 3 transient diabetes insipidus 1 permanent hypothalamic damage 2 transient trance-like states 1 transient 6th nerve weakness 1 slight permanent ptosis
Ziedses des Plantes and Creze	1978	61	
Vries	1978	5	
		236	4 transient oculomotor weaknesses 2 infections 1 subdural hydroma 2 transient mid-brain dysfunctions 4 transient hypothalamic damages 1 permanent hypothalamic damage

From the outset of this work, one of our concerns was the fear that, sooner or later, the communication between the third ventricle and the interpeduncular cistern would become obstructed. Indeed this happened: the recurrence rate was not negligible: 16.3%. However, it should be stressed that every time a second ventriculostomy was performed, it was successful.

One problem has been especially difficult with ventriculocisternostomies: how to estimate the results. In other words how to follow up the patients immediately after surgery, or months and years later. Early follow-up is most important since, if the ventriculocisternostomy is a failure, a valve should be inserted. We think that monitoring intracranial pressure (ICP) is the best way to check the efficiency of the ventriculocisternostomy. However, ICP should be recorded several times in the first 20 days after surgery because it returns to normal only gradually. That slow return towards normal proves that the subarachnoid spaces open up only progressively; it explains that isotope studies performed too early after surgery may give misleading results. It also shows that it is useless to insert a shunt prior to ventriculocisternostomy.

Another problem is to estimate the final result: Measuring head circumferences is disappointing since head circumference remains usually 2 or 3 SD above normal. On the other hand, no craniosynostosis was observed. Measuring the ventricular size is still more disappointing since some degree of dilatation persists after an initial decrease. However, we think that this dilatation is due to the slight persistent increase of the head circumference and does not imply any degree of atrophy. Finally, the best way to estimate the results of ventriculocisternostomies is to evaluate these children's IQs. IQ increases when ventriculocisternostomy is successful. The final result is statistically better or at least equal to the result achieved after insertion of a valve. In our series of ventriculocisternostomies, 82% of the patients have an IQ superior or equal to 80. These data demonstrate that, in spite of a persisting ventricular enlargement, IQs are good and that there is, in these children, no normal pressure hydrocephalus.

Returning to my first question: 'Are extracranial shunts the only surgical treatment in all cases of hydrocephalus?', my answer would be 'no' since percutaneous ventriculostomies can be proposed, as a first surgical procedure, in cases of non-communicating hydrocephalus in infants and children when the third ventricle is sufficiently dilated.

References

1 Brocklehurst, G.: Trans-callosal third ventriculo-chiasmatic cisternostomy: a new approach to hydrocephalus. Surg. Neurol. *2:* 109–114 (1974).

2 Dandy, W.E.: Extirpation of the choroid plexus of the lateral ventricle in communicating hydrocephalus. Ann. Surg. *68:* 569 (1918).

3 Dandy, W.E.: An operative procedure for hydrocephalus. Bull. Johns Hopkins Hosp. *33:* 189–190 (1922).

4 Dandy, W.E.: Surgery of the brain; in Lewis, Practice of surgery (Prior, Hagerstown (1932).

5 Davidoff, L.: Hydrocephalus and hydrocephalus with meningocele: their treatment by choroid plexectomy. Surg. Clins N. Am. *28:* 416 (1948).

6 Feld, M.; Ventriculoscope coagulant utilisé dans les hydrocéphalies communicantes. Presse, méd. *64:* 623 (1956).

7 Feld, N.: La coagulation des plexus choroides par ventriculoscopie directe dans l'hydrocéphalie non obstructive du nourrisson. Neuro-Chirurgie *3:* 70 (1957).

8 Forjaz, S.; Martelli, N.; Latuf, N.: Hypothalamic ventriculostomy with cathether. Technical note. J. Neurosurg. *29:* 655–659 (1968).

9 Guillaume, J.M.: L'ouverture de la lame sus-optique, traitement de certains dilatations ventriculaires. Press méd. *49:* 500–502 (1941).

10 Guillaume, J.M.; Mazars, G.: Indications et résultats de la ventriculostomie sus-optique dans l'hydrocéphalie de l'adulte. Revue neurol. *82:* 421–424 (1950).

11 Guiot, G.; Rougerie, J., Fourestier, M.; Fournier, A.; A.; Comoy, C.; Vulmiere, J.; Groux, R.: Explorations endoscopiques intra-crâniennes. Presse méd. *71:* 1224–1228 (1963).

12 Guiot, G.; Derome, P.; Hertzog, E.; Bamberger, C.; Akerman, M.: Ventriculo-cisternostomie sous contrôle radioscopique pour hydrocéphalie obstructive. Presse méd. *40:* 1923–1926 (1968).

13 Guiot, G.: Ventriculo-cisternostomy for stenosis of the aqueduct of Sylvius. Acta neurochir. *28:* 274–289 (1973).

14 Hirsch, J.F.; Renier, D.; Pierre-Kahn, A.; Lepintre, J.: Problèmes actuels dans la chirurgie de l'hydrocéphalie non-tumorale du nourrisson. Med. Inf. *4:* 369–381 (1976).

15 Hoffman, H.J.: The advantages of percutaneous third ventriculostomy over other forms of surgical treatment of infantile obstructive hydrocephalus; in Morley, Controversies in neurosurgery, pp. 691-703 (Saunders, Baltimore 1974).

16 Hyndman, O.R.: Hydrocephalus. A contribution related to treatment. J. Neurosurg. *3:* 426–443 (1946).

17 Lapras, C.; Poirier, N.; Deruty, R.; Bret, P.; Joyeux, O.: Le cathetérisme de l'aqueduc de Sylvius. Sa place actuelle dans le traitement chirurgical des sténoses de l'aqueduc de Sylvius, des tumeurs de la fosse cérébrale postérieure et de la syringomyélie. Neuro-Chirurgie *21:* 101–109 (1975).

18 Lapras, C.: Les sténoses de l'aqueduc de Sylvius. Rapport du XXXème Congr. Annuel de Neurochirurgie de Langue Française de 1980. Neuro-Chirurgie *26:* suppl., p. 153 (1980).

19 Lazorthes, G.; Anduze-Acher, H.; Campan, L.; Espagno, La ventriculo-cisternostomie transcalleuse: 4 ans d'expérience; 50 cas opérés. Neuro-Chirurgie *3:* 59–64 (1957).

20 Leksell, L.: A surgical procedure for atresia of the aqueduct of Sylvius. Acta psychiat. *24:* 559–569 (1949).

21 McNickle, H.F.: The surgical treatment of hydrocephalus. A simple method of performing third ventriculostomy. Br. J. Surg. *34:* 302–307 (1947).

22 Mixter, W.J.: Ventriculoscopy and puncture of the floor of the third ventricle. Preliminary report of a case. Boston med. Surg. J. *188:* 277–278 (1923).

23 Nulsen, F.E.; Spitz, E.B.: Treatment of hydrocephalus by direct shunt from ventricle to jugular vein. Surg. Forum *2:* 399–403 (1952).

24 Pierre-Kahn, A.; Renier, D.; Bombois, B.; Askienay, S.; Moreau, R.; Hirsch, J.F.: Place de la ventriculo-cisternostomie dans le traitement des hydrocéphalies non communicantes. Neuro-Chirurgie *21:* 557–559 (1975).

25a Putman, T.J.: Treatment of hydrocephalus by endoscopic coagulation of choroid plexuses: description of a new instrument. New Engl. J. Med. *210:* 1373 (1934).

25b Riechert quoted by Hemmer, R.: Der Hydrocephalus. Zbl. Neurochir. *12:* 36–46; 108–118 (1952).

26 Sachs, E.: Hydrocephalus: analysis of ninety-eight cases. J. Mt Sinai Hosp. *9:* 767 (1942).

27 Sayers, M.P.; Kosnick, E.J.: Percutaneous third ventriculostomy: experience and technique. Child's Brain *2:* 24–30 (1976).

28 Scarff, J.E.: Endoscopic treatment of hydrocephalus: description of a ventriculoscope and preliminary report of cases. Archs neurol. Psychiat., Chicago., *38:* 853–886 (1936).
29 Scarff, J.E.: Nonobstructive hydrocephalus: treatment by endoscopic cauterization of choroid plexus. Am. J. Dis. Child. *63:* 287 (1942).
30 Scarff, J.E.: Treatment of nonobstructive (communicating) hydrocephalus by cauterization of choroid plexuses: long-term follow-up study. Acta psychiat. scand. *34:* 354 (1959).
31 Scarff, J.E.: Evaluation of treatment of hydrocephalus. Results of third ventriculostomy and endoscopic cauterization of choroid plexuses compared with mechanical shunts. Archs Neurol., Chicago *14:* 382–391 (1966).
32 Stookey, B.; Scarff, J.E.: Occlusion of the aqueduct of Sylvius by neoplastic processes with a rational surgical treatment for relief of the resultant obstructive hydrocephalus. Bull. Neurol. Inst. N.Y. *5:* 348–377 (1936).
33 Torkildsen, A.: A new palliative operation in cases of inoperable occlusion of the Sylvian aqueduct. Acta chir. scand. *82:* 117–124 (1939).
34 Vries, J.K.: An endoscopic technique for third ventriculostomy. Surg. Neurol. *9:* 165–168 (1978).
35 White, J.C.; Michelsen, J.J.: Treatment of obstructive hydrocephalus in adults. Surgery Gynec. Obstet. *74:* 99–109 (1942).
36 Williams, B.: Is aqueduct stenosis a result of hydrocephalus? Brain *96:* 399–412 (1973).
37 Ziedses des Plantes, B.G.; Crezee, P.: Transfrontal perforation of the lamina terminalis. Neuroradiology *16:* 51–53 (1978).

Prof. J.-F. Hirsch Hôpital Necker Enfants-Malades, 149 rue des Sèvres
F–75730 Paris Cedex 15 (France)

Monogr. neural Sci., vol. 8, pp. 179–183 (Karger, Basel 1982)

Hydrodynamics of Shunts

Harold D. Portnoy[1]

Departments of Health Sciences and Physics, Oakland University, Rochester, Mich., Department of Surgery (Neurosurgery), Crittenton Hospital, Rochester, Mich., USA

What are the most desirable pressure-flow characteristics of a shunt? Several neurosurgeons have commented that the ideal valve should be flow-controlled. Such a valve would have to continuously determine the formation rate and the rate of outflow through natural channels, and regulate the flow through the valve so as to remove only the excess fluid. There is no mechanism now available that can accomplish this without difficulty, much less be capsuled into a volume of 3 ml or less. Thus, it is necessary to use the present pressure-regulated devices which attempt to maintain a predetermined ventricular fluid pressure (VFP).

Silicone rubber slit valves maintain a given VFP poorly for two reasons: (1) the pressure at the inlet of the valve varies greatly depending on the flow through the valve, and (2) the pressure-flow curve of the valve varies depending on whether the valve has been recently irrigated or allowed to rest. These problems are illustrated in figure 1. As flow varies from 0.2 to 0.6 $ml \cdot min^{-1}$, the range found in patients undergoing CSF hydrodynamic testing [4, 5], the inlet pressure of the valve may vary 3- to 4-fold. In addition, as noted in figure 1 the pressure-flow characteristics of slit valves vary with the pretreatment of the valve [2] so that the difference at a given formation rate (e.g. 0.35 $ml \cdot min^{-1}$) may be significant.

Hakim et al. [3] noted that the ideal pressure-regulating device should have a rapid run off of fluid once open. As illustrated in figure 2, two types of valves have this characteristic, the spring-ball valve and the silicone rubber diaphragm valve. ASTM Standards were followed in testing of shunt components [1]. Both maintain a fairly constant inlet pressure even at high flow rates as long as the outlet is kept at atmospheric pressure and no other valve is in the shunt system. Unfortunately neither one of these two conditions may actually exist.

[1] The author appreciates the technical assistance of Mr. *R. Redmond.*

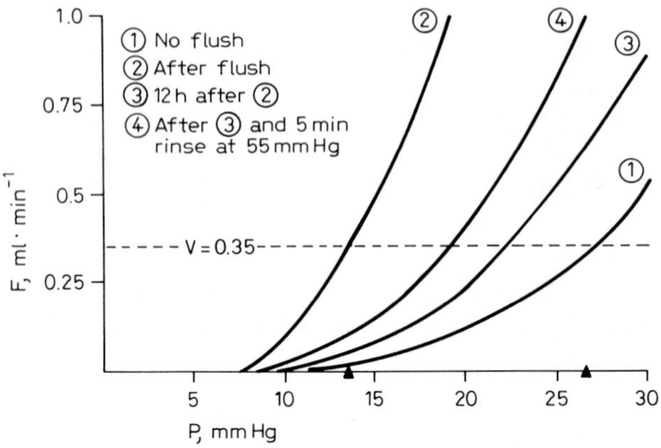

Fig. 1. Pressure-flow data from a silicone rubber slit valve (medium pressure). Note the marked variation in pressure at various flow rates. In particular, note that the shape of the curve is markedly dependent on the pretreatment of the valve [adapted from 2]. V- formation rate.

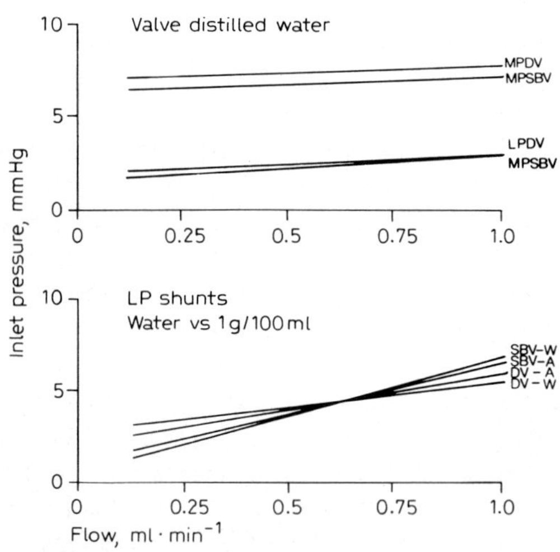

Fig. 2. Pressure-flow data from spring-ball and silicone rubber diaphragm valves. Note that a marked variation in flow produces only a small change in pressure. Both have virtually the same characteristics when irrigated with water or 1g/100 mg albumin solution. Abbreviations for this and subsequent figures: LP = low-pressure; MP = medium pressure; SBV = spring-ball valve; SVC = slit valve catheter; ASD = antisiphon device; W = water; A = albumin.

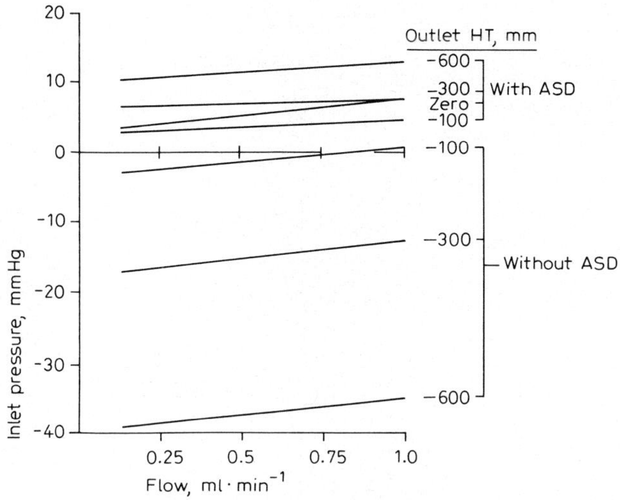

Fig. 3. Presure-flow data from a shunt composed of a low-pressure spring-ball valve and low-pressure distal slit valve catheter. Lowering of the distal catheter by 100, 300, and 600 mm results in markedly negative inlet pressures even at a flow rate of 1.0 ml • min $^{-1}$. addition of an ASD eliminates the negative pressure.

The pressure at the outlet of the valve is significantly affected by the attached distal catheter. If the end of the catheter is below the valve outlet a negative pressure is produced which when measured in mm H_2O is equal to the vertical height of the catheter. This will reduce the effective opening pressure of the valve or keep the valve open and draining continuously. In figure 3 is presented the pressure-flow data of a low-pressure spring-ball valve and low-pressure slit valve catheter which was irrigated at between 0.1 and 1.0 ml • min^{-1}. The inlet pressure varied between 3.5 and 7 mm Hg. The tip of the catheter was then lowered by 100, 300, and 600 mm simulating what would happen if a patient stood up from a reclining position. The inlet (ventricular) pressure dropped, reaching as low as –40 mm Hg. By adding an antisiphon device (ASD) immediatly at the valve outlet, the negative pressure produced by the siphoning effect of the distal catheter was negated and the inlet pressure remained positive.

The ASD simply maintains the outlet pressure of the valve at approximately atmospheric pressure which is the condition under which the valve was calibrated. It should be remembered that the addition of an ASD reduces the overall daily flow through the valve by eliminating the siphon effect of the distal catheter. If the ASD is attached to an existing medium or high-pressure shunt it may result in inadequate shunting. The ASD alone does not significantly change the pressure-flow characteristics of the valve (fig. 5). It does, however, eliminate

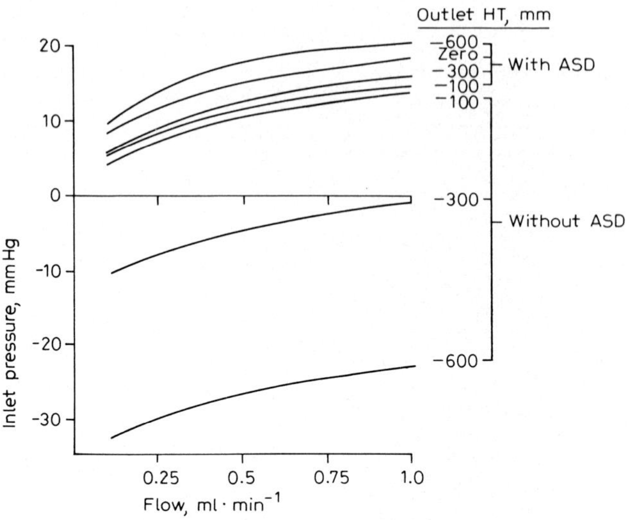

Fig. 4. Pressure-flow data from a shunt composed of a low-pressure slit valve and low-pressure distal slit valve catheter. This combination results in higher inlet pressures at all flow rates. Siphoning helps reduce the higher pressures to acceptable levels. The ASD tends to accentuate the higher pressures.

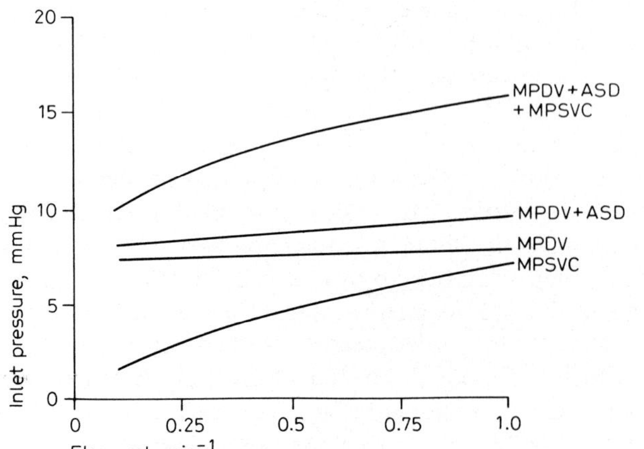

Fig. 5. Pressure-flow data from a medium-pressure diaphragm valve, medium-pressure slit valve catheter, and ASD. Note that the resistance of a shunt (measured as pressure/flow or mm Hg · ml^{-1} · min) is equal to the sum of the resistances of its component parts.

the flow through the valve due to siphoning. Particularly with some slit valves, adequate flow is maintained by utilizing the siphon effect. In these instances, the addition of an ASD may result in inadequate shunting (fig. 4). In contrast, spring-ball and diaphragm valves yield very low pressures when the patient stands and are stabilized by the addition of an ASD (fig. 3).

Another pitfall in shunt implantation is the presence of two valves in series. Usually only one of the two valves is looked upon as the control valve and the existence of the other valve virtually ignored. The resistances of valves in series are additive. As demonstrated in figure 5, when a medium-pressure distal slit valve is added to a medium-pressure proximal diaphragm valve the resultant is a high-pressure shunt with pressure-flow characteristics most resembling the slit valve. If pressure control is desired at the proximal valve then the distal slit valve catheter should be of a low-pressure type. It should have virtually no resistance to flow. A common error is connecting a medium-pressure proximal and a medium-pressure distal valve in series believing the end result is a medium-pressure shunt. Usually it is a high-pressure shunt. Such a shunt may work adequately without an ASD but fail with the device. The neurosurgeon usually condemns the ASD not realizing the complex valve system is a high-pressure shunt which should not contain an ASD.

The ideal shunt should consist of a spring-ball or diaphragm proximal valve of the desired pressure range, an ASD to stabilize the valve, and a low-pressure distal slit valve catheter so as not to alter the desirable characteristics of the proximal valve.

References

1 American Society for Testing and Materials Standards F 647–79. Standard practice for the evaluation and specification of implantable shunt assemblies for neurosurgical application.

2 Ekstedt, J.; Friden, H.: Hydrodynamic properties of CSF shunt systems; in Shulman, Marmarou, Miller, Hochwald, Brock, Intracranial pressure IV, pp. 483–488 (Springer, Berlin, 1980).

3 Hakim, S., Roche, F.D. de la; Burton, J.D.: A critical analysis of valve shunts used in the treatment of hydrocephalus. Devl Med. Child Neurol. *15:* 230–255 (1973).

4 Portnoy, H.D.; Croissant, P.D.: Pre- and postoperative cerebrospinal fluid absorption studies in patients with myelomeningocele shunted for hydrocephalus. Child's Brain *4:* 47–64 (1978).

5 Portnoy, H.D.; Croissant, P.D.: Megalencephaly in infants and children. The possible role of increased dural sinus pressure. Archs Neurol., Chicago *35:* 306–316 (1978).

H.D. Portnoy, MD, Oakland Neurological Clinic, 1431 Woodward,
Bloomfield Hills, MI 48013 (USA)

Monogr. neural Sci., vol. 8, pp. 184–187 (Karger, Basel 1982)

How to Choose the Best Valve

F. Buchheit, D. Maitrot, J.L. Healy, S. Gusmao
Pavillon Clovis Vincent, Hôpital Civil, Strasbourg, France

Measurement of the Differential Pressure

We can compare a shunt and its valve (slit or ball-valve) to a derivation between two tanks. The working of the valve does not depend only on the proximal tank's pressure but on the differential pressure (DP) between the proximal and the distal tanks (fig. 1). This DP is equal to: DP = PA–PB, where PA is the pressure just above the valve and PB, the pressure just after the valve.

$$PA = PO + P1 + l1,$$
$$PB = PO + P2 - l2,$$
$$DP = (PO + P1 + l1) - (PO + P2 - L2),$$
$$= P1 + (l1 + l2) - P2,$$
$$= P1 + L - P2,$$

where P1 is the ICP, L is the length of the shunt, P2 is the intra-atrial pressure or intra-abdominal pressure (IAP), and DP = ICP + L–IAP. Are we able to know the mean value of these three parameters?

ICP. For the hydrocephalic child, without shunt, the ICP varies usually between 80 and 150 mm H_2O, whatever his position. For the non-hydrocephalic child, the ICP varies between –70 mm H_2O in the erect position and plus 100 mm H_2O in the lying position. For the hydrocephalic child with shunt, the ICP varies according to the position of the child and the type of the valve and of the shunt. *MacCullough and Fox* [4] report pressures from –250 to –440 mm H_2O for hydrocephalic patients with shunt.

Length of the shunt. This is very easy to measure. It depends upon the age of the child and his length, and varies between 120 and 800 mm. It is always zero in the lying position.

Intra-atrial or intra-abdominal pressure is also known. For a VC shunt, IAP equals zero or is slightly negative in the lying and erect position. For a VP shunt in the erect position, IAP depends on the exact position of the end of the

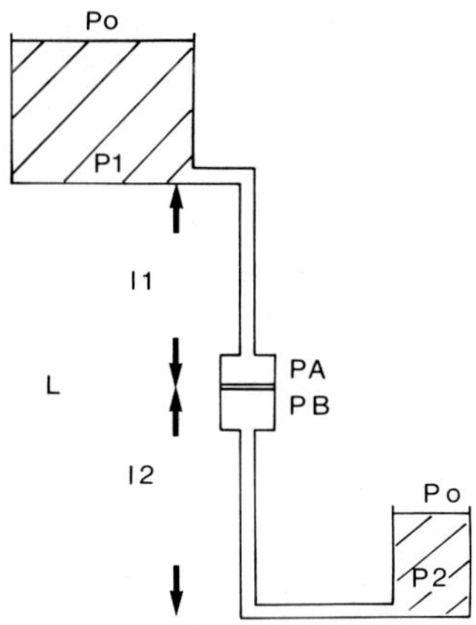

Fig. 1. PO = Atmospheric pressure; P1 = proximal reservoir pressure; P2 = distal reservoir pressure; PA = pressure in front of the valve; PB = pressure after the valve; l1 = height of proximal catheter; l2 = height of distal catheter; L = length of shunt (l1 + l2). P1 = ICP (intracranial pressure); P2 = IAP (intra-atrial or intra-abdominal pressure).

peritoneal catheter: (1) zero in the inter-hepato-diaphragmatic position; (2) 150 mm H_2O on the level of the navel for adult, between 80 and 150 mm H_2O for children equalizing the distance between the diaphragm and the navel, and (3) 300 mm H_2O on the level of the Douglas pouch. For a VP shunt in the lying position, IAP is always 80 mm H_2O in all the abdominal cavity. Knowing the DP for a valve, we are also able to settle the flow rate of the valve.

Flow Rates of the Valves

Forrest [1] and *Potthoff and Hemmer* [6] ascertain numerous differences between the valves concerning their flow rates.

How to measure the flow rates of the valves. We use a reservoir of 17 cm diameter and 8.5 cm high (fig. 1). The issue of the reservoir has a diameter of 1.2 mm, that is the diameter of the catheter of the shunts. This reservoir is big enough to obtain no significant variation in the level of the water during the test.

All the valves were tested according to the instructions of the manufacturer. The DP is measured according to our equation explained before, that is DP = P1 + L–P2. We measure, then, the volume of water which flowed during the test and this for several DPs and each time for three valves of the same kind. The results are seen in figure 2 and concern: Holter valves, Holter-Hausner valves, Hakim valves, the Denver valve, and the unishunt of Codman, being the valves we use in the service.

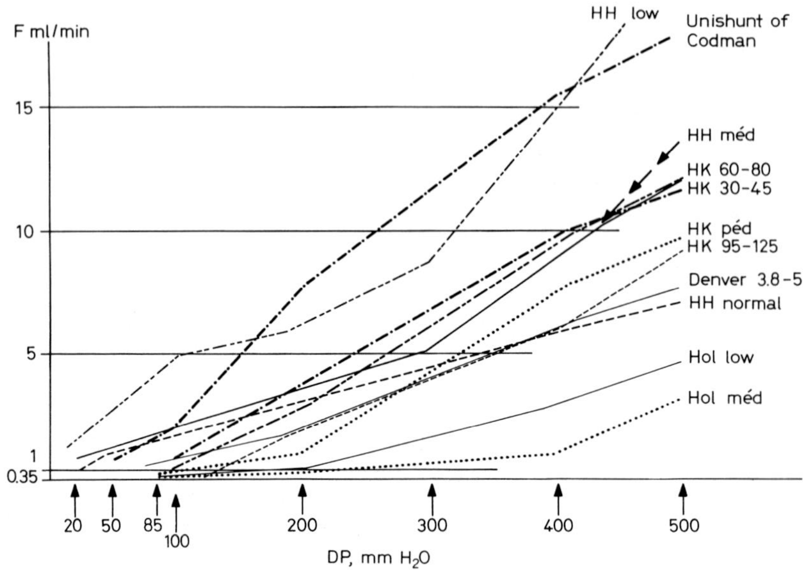

Fig. 2. Flow rates of the valves according to the DP. The physiological flow rate of CSF (0.35 ml/min) is shown on the first line.

Discussion

High variations of flow rate exist for the same DP according to the type of valve. For example: Holter (extracorporeal) valves have low flow rates which are less than the normal flow rate of CSF as long as the DP is lower than 200 mm H_2O. Hakim valves have a flow rate much greater, but near the normal flow rate of CSF between 85 and 130 mm H_2O of DP according to the type of valve. These two kinds of valves do not work if the DP is less than 85 mm H_2O. The flow rate of the Denver valve (3.8–5 ml) is the same as the Hakim valve (95–125 mm H_2O) except for the low DP where the flow rate remains over the normal flow of CSF. The flow rates of Holter-Hausner valves are very high whatever the DP is, particularly for the lowest DP. This means that the valves stay invariably opened. The unishunt of Codman has a flow rate near the Holter-Hausner low-pressure valve. The obstacles produced by the latter valves is so small that they are only to by regarded as derivations.

Choice of the Valve

Because we do not know the flow rate of CSF in each hydrocephalus, we state that a valve whose flow rate is the nearest of the physiological one is to be used. So, after measuring the exact DP for a child, we can choose the best valve. Before giving an example, we have to keep in mind that, in the lying position: (1) for a VA shunt, DP = ICP; (2) for a VP shunt, DP = ICP −80 mm H_2O.

Example. Case of a VA procedure at birth: L = 130 for VC shunt; L = 230 for VP shunt in the erect position. If we want a valve working in a lying position, it is an ICP of less than 100 mm H_2O which is alone responsible for the flow rate. We have then to choose a Holter-Hausner valve or a unishunt. But in the erect position, ICP becomes negative and the factor L grows from zero to 130. The flow rate of this valve will remain higher than necessary, or perhaps too high, and a ventricular collapse can appear. This is why, in the lying position, we prefer a valve whose flow rate is smaller for the usual DP (100 mm H_2O and less), for example the Hakim 60–80. In these conditions, when the child is in the sitting position, if we argue as previously, for an ICP near zero and a length of tube of 130 mm, we get flow rates near the physiological one.

Conclusions

According to our equation DP = ICP + L–IAP, we try to choose the best valve. Usually, for low DP (less than 200 mm H_2O; fig. 2), we can use many kinds of valves but those whose flow rates are near the physiological one are to be preferred. Over 200 mm H_2O of DP, the best choice, it seems to us, is the Holter (extracorporeal) valve.

References

1 Forrest, D.M.: Flow characteristics of the Spitz-Holter valve. Devl Med. Child Neurol. *4:* 295–297 (1962).

2 Forrest, D.M.; Cooper, D.G.W.: Complications of ventriculo-atrial shunts; a review of 455 cases. J. Neurosurg. *29:* 506–513 (1968).

3 Gusmao, S.: Etude expérimentale de l'hydrodynamique des valves et son application clinique. A propos de 107 cas (Mémoire, Strasbourg 1979).

4 MacCullough, D.C., Fox, J.L.: Negative intracranial pressure hydrocephalus in adults with shunts and its relationship to the production of subdural hematoma. J. Neurosurg. *40:* 372–375 (1974).

5 MacCullough, D.C.; Fox, J.L.; Curl, F.; Green, R.C.: Effect of CSF shunts on intracranial pressure and CSF dynamics; in Harbert, Cisternography and hydrocephalus, pp. 335–342 (Thomas , Springfield 1972).

6 Potthoff, P.C.; Hemmer, R.: Valve insufficiency in ventriculo-atrial shunts. Devl Med. Child Neurol. *20:* suppl., p. 38 (1969).

F. Buchheit, MD, Pavillon Clovis Vincent, Hôpital Civil, Strasbourg (France)

Monogr. neural Sci., vol. 8, pp. 188–190 (Karger, Basel 1982)

Evaluation and Use of the Once-Piece and Three-Piece Ventriculoperitoneal Shunts in Infantile Hydrocephalus

F. Castellanos, R. Guillen, S. Martinez-Lirio, J. Jimenez-Castellanos
Neurosurgical Service of the University Hospital (Prof. *Jimenez-Castellanos*), University Medical School, Seville, Spain

Introduction

One of the most important problems that neurosurgery has planned is the surgical treatment of hydrocephalus, showing several different methods and surgical techniques in order to elude the numerous complications that the external shunting systems present. At present we think that ventriculoperitoneal shunting is a better start of treatment in infantile hydrocephalus, so in this report we make only a critical comparative study between two different methods of ventriculoperitoneal shunting: the one-piece (Raimondi's unishunt) and the three-piece (Holter's system) shunts. Data are presented descriptively, as an analysis of possible complications. Finally we discuss the advantages and disadvantages of both shunting systems according to our personal experience [1, 2].

Clinical Material and Methods

In this work we study the results of the surgical treatment of 52 children with congenital or acquired hydrocephalus by means of the one-piece and three-piece ventriculoperitoneal shunting systems, in the Neurosurgical Service of the University Hospital of Seville, Spain. We have reviewed our series of the last 5 years (January 1975 to January 1980), with 168 hydrocephalus in total, in which two groups of 26 hydrocephalic children have been selected by hazard and treated with the one-piece and three-piece systems, respectively, and in whom a total of 76 surgical procedures, removals and/or revisions were realized. The etiology of our cases is the following: obstructive hydrocephalus, 23; communicating hydrocephalus, 9; myelomeningocele, 10, and tumors, 10.

The patients ranged in age between 2 days and 14 years, with an average about 3 years and distributed as follows: 0–1 months, 12; 1–3 months, 6; 3–12 months, 4; 1–2 years, 7; 2–4 years, 9; 4–10 years, 10, and 10–14 years, 4. The follow-up of these cases oscillated between 58 and 3 months, with an average of 27 months. The Holter's shunts used were classified according to pressure: extra low, 3; low, 19, and medium, 4. A high-pressure shunt was never used. All the unishunts used were of 2–5 cm H_2O pressure and their lengths ranged between 53 and 78 cm according to age and length of the patients. The peritoneal catheter was always introduced through a split trocar [3] as a pararentesis puncture, without any complications.

Results

The general results of the 52 hydrocephalic children are distributed as follows: 26 unishunts with 17 patients without complications and 9 with complications in whom 11 removals were made, twice in 2 patients. 26 Holter's systems with 16 patients without complications and 10 with complications in whom 13 surgical procedures were made, twice in 3 cases.

The total complications were 27, divided in 16 for Holter's systems and 11 for unishunts, distributed as follows: obstruction, 9 in Holter's and 2 in unishunts; infection, 4 and 3; intolerance, 2 and 2, and emigration, 1 and 4, respectively.

The removals were as follows: (a) Holter's system: ventricular catheter, 5 cases; shunting valve, 2 cases. Distal catheter, 1 case, equal system, 2 cases, and another system, 3 cases, divided in 1 low atrial Holter's system, 1 removal of the shunting system and 1 unishunt. (b) Unishunt systems: catheter reposition (cephalic end), 2 cases; obstruction, intolerance, 4 cases; changes to a similar system, 2 cases; and changes to another system, 3 cases (3 low Holter's systems).

Discussion

Summarizing these results we can study, in relation with each type of ventriculoperitoneal shunting, the evolution time for the first removal, average number of complications per patient and surgical procedure and, finally, we analyze these complications divided into four groups: obstruction, infection, intolerance, and emigration.

First, we have verified that 50% of the complications were produced during the first 3 months following insertion of the shunting system, to reach almost 70% of the cases in the one-piece shunts. In relation with the total complications and rate per patient, our results were almost the same in each group with 38 and 35%, respectively, in the three-piece and one-piece shunting systems, without any significant difference by means of the χ^2 statistical test.

Similarly comparing total complications to surgical procedures shows that, in the one-piece series, 26 cases with 11 complications in 9 children (30%) and a total of 37 operations offers a procedure mean per child of 1.4, lower than the 1.9 of *Raimondi et al.* [4], and higher than the 1.1 of *Villarejo et al.* [5], but very like the mean obtained in our three-piece series of 26 patients with 13 complications (33%) in 10 cases and 39 operations, with an average per child of 1.5; the results are without any statistical significance. However, if we analyze these results for each complication, it is noteworthy that, in relation with the obstruction series, there is an incidence in 23% of the three-piece cases, a complication rate almost four times higher than the 6% incidence of obstruction in the one-piece series, a difference with statistical significance ($\chi^2 = 4.94$, $p < 0.05$) that permits us to realize in conclusion the advantage of the one-piece shunt in relation with this complication.

The other series of complications, as infection, whose frequency in our cases is lowest (10 and 8% against 16 and 11% of the series of *Raimondi et al.* [4], intolerance (5% in both series), and slipping or disconnection (3 and 11%), there is no statistical significance to make our choice for one of these shunt types, although in the last complication series of emigration we like to show that in our opinion the apparent difference appeared to be due to the influence of a correct surgical technique in order to avoid disconnection in the three-piece system and, also in our experience, was owed to the fixation system of the unishunt by clips, because in the 4 cases of peritoneal end emigration, 2 of the cerebral ventricle and 2 of the peritoneal cavity, with total introduction of 1 of them into the cerebral ventricle, the surgical revision showed that the security clips were correctly closed.

To resume, our personal experience shows that if we excluded the higher incidence of obstruction in the three-piece shunts, logically by the connections and shunting valve, there is no statistically significant difference between the one-piece systems regarding results and complications; although by its better, easy, and rapid surgical implantation and its lower obstructive frequency, we prefer the use of the one-piece shunting system, especially in the first 6 months of life.

References

1 Castellanos Mateos, F.; Guillen Quesada, R.; Martinez Lirio, S.; Jimenez-Castellanos, J.: Estudio comparativo de los shunts ventriculoperitoneales de una y tres piezas en el tratamiento quirurgico de las hidrocefalias infantiles. Comunicación a la XXXII Reunión de la Sociedad Luso-Española de Neurocirugía, Oporto 1980.

2 Lajat, Y.; Lebatard-Sartre, R.; Guihard, D.; Ito, I.; Fresche, F.; Collet, M.; Descuns, P.: Etude comparative des complications observées dans les dérivations ventriculoatriales et ventriculopéritonéales. Neuro-Chirurgie *21:* 147–161 (1965).

3 Raimondi, A.J.: Ventriculoperitoneal shunting. A technique for inserting the one-piece shunt. Signatures series 6 (Codman, Randolph 1975).

4 Raimondi, A.J.; Robinson, J.S.; Kuwamura, K.: Complications of ventriculoperitoneal shunting and a critical comparison of the three-piece and one-piece systems. Child's Brain *3:* 321–342 (1977).

5 Villarejo, F.; Heredero, J.; Amaya, C.: Hydrodephalus in children treated with the one-piece shunt. Child's Brain *4:* 360–364 (1978).

F. Castellanos, MD, Neurosurgical Service of the University Hospital,
University Medical School, Seville (Spain)

Monogr. neural Sci., vol. 8, pp. 191–194 (Karger, Basel 1982)

Floating Ventricular Catheter: A New Shunting Device

Saburo Nakamura, Nobuo Moriyasu

Department of Neurosurgery, School of Medicine Nihon University, Tokyo, Japan

Among various complications after ventriculostomy, obstruction of the shunting system has been reported to have the most frequent occurrence [1, 5, 7, 9, 10]. In the paper of *Steinbok and Thompson* [8], 289 out of 503 ventriculo-atrial (VA) shunted cases had complications and 130 of these 289 cases of complications had malfunction of the shunting system. Of the 130 patients, dysfunction of the ventricular catheter was recognized in 86 (66%). In another report by *Illingworth et al.* [4], of 71 complications, disturbance of the ventricular cathether was reported in 31, that is 42.7%. *Forrest and Cooper* [2] presented 147 revisions due to dysfunction of the ventricular catheter in a total of 455 VA shunted patients. The most frequent cause leading to the dysfunction was obstruction by the choroid plexus, which was found 74 times, that is in 50.3%. All of the papers mentioned reported that complications due to obstruction of the ventricular catheter showed the highest occurrence, and obstruction by the choroid plexus was the most frequent.

Floating Ventricular Catheter

A new ventricular catheter has been designed to prevent such obstruction by the choroid plexus or the ventricular wall. This new catheter is characterized by its floatation, by means of an air cell attached to the distal end of the catheter (fig. 1). The air cell is 16 mm long, with a 1.6-mm lumen and 2.4-mm outside diameter, and is connected to the leading catheter, which is 1.7 mm in outside diameter. A black line on the air cell which is visible by X-ray examination acts as a marker. At the end of the leading catheter there are four small holes, 0.6 mm in diameter, which serve as inlets via which CSF enters. The flowing volume through the catheter in relation to pressure is shown in figure 2. The flowing volume is, for example, as much as 3.65 ml/min at a pressure of 100 mm H_2O.

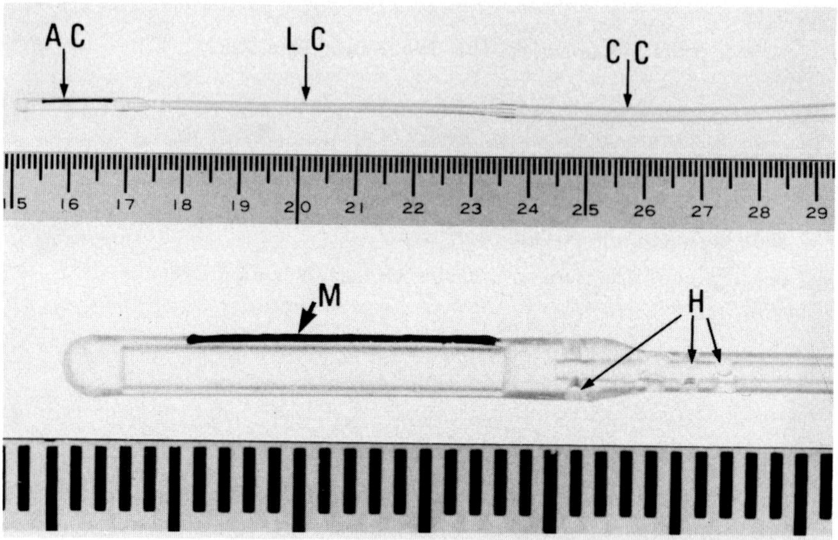

Fig. 1. Floating ventricular catheter. AC = Air cell; CC = connecting catheter; H = hole; LC = leading catheter; M = marker.

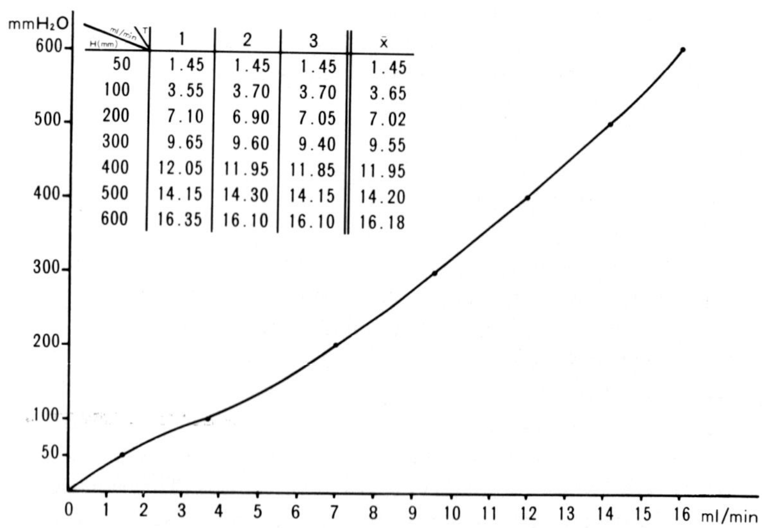

H(mm) \ ml/min, T	1	2	3	x̄
50	1.45	1.45	1.45	1.45
100	3.55	3.70	3.70	3.65
200	7.10	6.90	7.05	7.02
300	9.65	9.60	9.40	9.55
400	12.05	11.95	11.85	11.95
500	14.15	14.30	14.15	14.20
600	16.35	16.10	16.10	16.18

Fig. 2. Flowing volume through the catheter in relation to pressure.

Results

The catheter has so far been used in 14 cases, 2 of whom died at 5 and 9 months after operation due to pneumonia and peritonitis, respectively. In 1 patient, the catheter had to be removed at 5 months after ventriculostomy due to infection of the shunting system. However, in the other 11 cases the system has functioned well for over 19 months since surgery, the longest time interval being 37 months. No trouble due to shunt function has yet been encountered. In the 3 cases where shunting was interrupted, the ventricular catheter was clear and not plugged by the choroid plexus or cerebral debris.

Discussion

As regards the obstruction mechanism of the ventricular catheter, the following three factors can be considered: (1) plugging by the choroid plexus, (2) plugging by cerebral debris as the dilated ventricle becomes reduced in size after ventricular shunt, and (3) capture in the choroid plexus as a foreign body reaction.

Several new shunting catheters have been devised to prevent obstruction of the ventricular catheter; for example, Portnoy's flanged tip catheter [6], Garner's balloon catheter [3], the multi-pored flange catheter [3], and Carrea's cage catheter [3]. These catheters were designed so as to avoid plugging by the choroid plexus or cerebral debris, by maintaining a distance between the inlet of the catheter and choroid plexus or ventricular wall with a flange, balloon or cage. However, these catheters did not always function well and were caught by the choroid plexus. As experienced by many surgeons, once the catheter has become captured, to pull it out for revision is very difficult and dangerous due to the complicated shape of the catheter with its additional apparatus.

The floating ventricular catheter keeps its end on the opposite side against gravity, and when the catheter is inserted into the anterior horn, it maintains an effective distance between the catheter inlet and choroid plexus in any head position unless the patient is standing on his head. Furthermore, the slender and flexible leading catheter alters its position easily with head movement and is so able to avoid capture by the choroid plexus or ventricular wall.

References

1 Becker, D.P.; Nulsen, F.E.: Control of hydrocephalus by valve-regulated venous shunt: avoidance of complications in prolonged shunt maintenance. J. Neurosurg. *28:* 215–226 (1968).
2 Forrest, D.M.; Cooper, D.G.W.: Complications of ventriculoatrial shunts. J. Neurosurg. *29:* 506–512 (1968).

3 Garner, J.T.. Heyer-Schulte Corporation.
4 Illingworth, R.D.; Logue, V.; Symon, L.; Uemura, K.: The ventriculocaval shunt in the treatment of adult hydrocephalus: results and complications in 101 patients. J. Neurosurg. *35:* 681–685 (1971).
5 Little, J.R., Rhoton, A.L.Jr.; Mellinger, J.F.: Comparison of ventriculoperitoneal and ventriculoatrial shunts for hydrocephalus in children. Surg. Neurol. *5:* 31–35 (1976).
6 Portnoy, H.D.: New ventricular catheter for hydrocephalic shunts. Technical note. J. Neurosurg. *34:* 702–703 (1971).
7 Putman, T.J.: Surgical treatment of infantile hydrocephalus. Surgery Gynec. Obstet. *76:* 171–182 (1943).
8 Steinbok, P.; Thompson, G.B.: Complications of ventriculovascular shunts: computer analysis of etiological factors. Mayo Clin. Proc. *47:* 396–401 (1972).
9 Steinke, H.J.: Funktionstechnik und Komplikationsursachen bei ventrikuloatrialen Shunts. Zentbl. Neurochir. *28:* 203–215 (1968).
10 Stenger, L.: Complications of ventriculovenous shunts. J. Neurosurg. *20:* 219–224 (1963).

S. Nakamura, MD, Department of Neurosurgery, School of Medicine, Nihon University, Tokyo (Japan)

Monogr. neural Sci., vol. 8, pp. 195–198 (Karger, Basel 1982)

A Surgical Device Standard for Neurosurgical Shunt Assemblies

Larry K. Page

Division of Pediatric Neurosurgery, University of Miami, Miami, Fla., USA

The United States Government passed a law several years ago which requires its Federal Drug Administration (FDA) to assure the safety and efficacy of all implanted surgical devices. In anticipation of the passage of this law, the American Society for Testing and Materials (ASTM), a voluntary standards organization, undertook the writing of a standard for neurosurgical shunts. After 6 years of development, this became an official document in December 1979. The FDA now has available a standard method to evaluate new shunts and shunt components prior to release for marketing. If new products differ significantly from the Standard, extensive and rigorous pre-market testing will be necessary to evaluate them for use by the public.

The Standard [4] specifies types of materials, mechanical properties and surface finish that are currently acceptable in the manufacture of shunts. The best available tests that are necessary to assure biocompatibility of shunt materials are listed. The various component parts of a shunt system are defined. The minimal requirements for packaging, labeling and sterility of the products are specified. The recommended test method for determining radio-opacity of shunt components is described. Finally, the Standard recommends a particular test method for evaluating the pressure-flow characteristics of valves. It is the intent of the neurosurgeons, shunt manufacturers, engineers, and basic scientists who developed this Standard that it provide reasonable and useful guidelines to the government for assessing the safety and efficacy of new products and that it provide a common language to producers and users of these devices that they may be more easily and accurately described, and compared, to the ultimate benefit of the individual patient.

The specific terms in table I were chosen so that all currently available shunting device components could be readily described. Thus, the extracorporeal Holter system consists of a proximal catheter, a reservoir, two valves and a distal catheter. The Cordis-Hakim device consists of a proximal catheter, an ante-

Table I. Standard terms for the components of neurosurgical shunting devices

1	Proximal catheter (inflow)
2	Distal catheter (outflow)
3	Connector
4	Valve
5	Valved catheter
6	Implantable accessory device
	(a) Antechamber
	(b) Antisiphon
	(c) Flushing
	(d) In-line filter
	(e) On-off switch
	(f) Reservoir

chamber, two valves and a distal catheter. The Denver shunt combines a proximal catheter, a reservoir, a valve and a valved catheter. The Dow-Corning-Ames shunt has two flushing devices and a valved catheter. Heyer-Schulte offers several accessory devices that may be coupled with a valved catheter. The Codman-Raimondi unishunt consists of a one-piece combination of proximal catheter and valved catheter.

The test method for evaluation of the pressure-flow characteristics of neurosurgical shunt assemblies requires a source-fluid reservoir, a variable speed pump calibrated in ml/h, a water manometer calibrated in mm, a constant level water bath and the device to be tested. The test fluid and water bath temperatures must be held at 37°C. The test fluid medium is deaerated distilled water. All air is purged from the shunt system by irrigating with the test fluid at a pressure not to exceed 500 mm H_2O while the shunt is submerged in the water bath for a sufficient period of time to assure stable pressure-flow characteristics. The zero level of the manometer is at the fluid level of the water bath. The pump speed is adjusted and the manometer pressure level is recorded after stabilization, for at least five flow rates, down-ramping from 50 to 5 ml/h.

It is generally accepted that CSF production rates are relatively constant, approximately 0.35 ml/min or 20 ml/h in both normal and hydrocephalic patients [2]. However, CSF absorption rates vary directly with pressure. *Cutler et al.* [1] found that, in normal patients, at 20 ml/h mean production and absorption rates, CSF pressure is approximately 112 mm H_2O. However, the slope, or the threshold, of the regression line for absorption in hydrocephalic patients is increased [2, 3]. The pressure-flow slope of a shunting device, initially at least, should be less than the normal absorption slope.

The pressure-flow test method of this ASTM Standard was recently set up in our laboratory using a Harvard apparatus syringe pump. We randomly took one

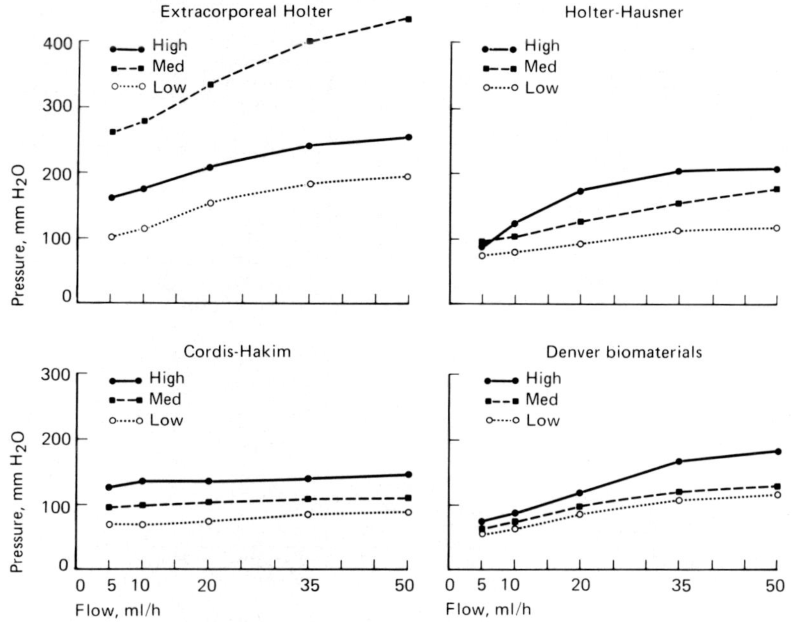

Fig. 1. Results of testing randomly selected devices by the ASTM standard method.

high, one medium, and one low shunt device produced by each US manufacturer from the storage shelves in our operating rooms and tested them in the prescribed manner. Since flow is the independent variable in this testing method, pressure becomes the dependent variable and is displayed on the ordinates in figures 1 and 2.

Although the Cordis Company uses ball valve mechanisms, the other US manufacturers currently depend upon nonporous polymeric slit valves. When not used, and especially when stored dry, silicone has a tendency to self-adhere. It is therefore important to manipulate or irrigate these valves in order to open them completely. They must then be allowed time to regain the elastic properties that are temporarily changed by distortion of the polymer.

The extracorporeal Holter slit valves are housed in metal and cannot be directly inspected and manipulated to ascertain that portions of the slits are not adhered. We have found that, after purging by up-ramping the flow rate to produce a pressure of 500 mm H_2O for 1 min, they should soak in the water bath for at least 4 h prior to testing.

The Standard does not require all of the manufacturers to use the same ranges for the high, medium and low groups. It does provide a standard test

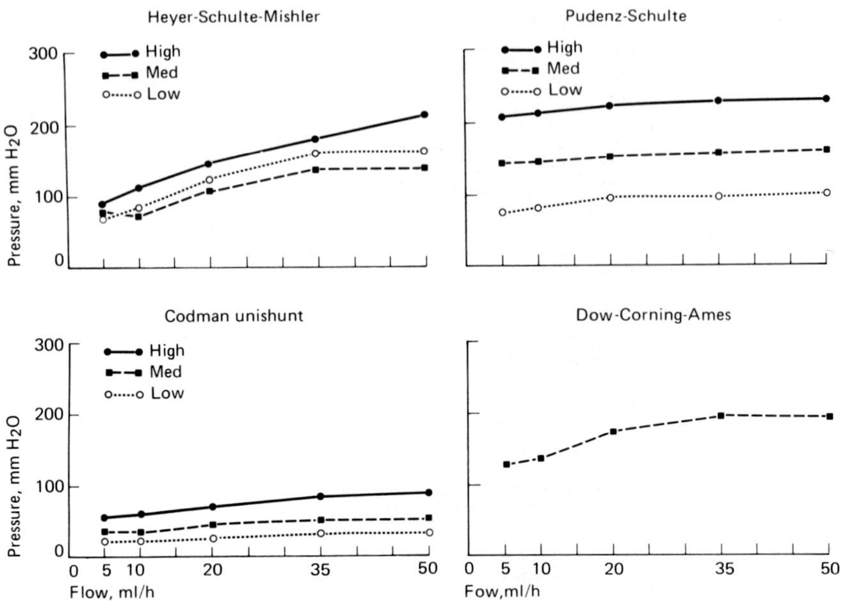

Fig. 2. Each plot is the test result for a single shunting device.

method and a standard reporting system. The manufacturers are free to choose whatever pressure-flow limits they wish for each group. However, they must then individually test each device to assure that it falls within its assigned pressure-flow range.

References

1 Cutler, R.W.P.; Page, L.K.; Galicich, J.H.; Watters, G.V.: Formation and absorption of CSF in man. Brain *91:* 707–720 (1968).

2 Lorenzo, A.V.; Page, L.K.; Watters, G.V.: Relationship between CSF formation and pressure in human hydrocephalus. Brain *93:* 679–692 (1970).

3 Page, L.K.; Bresnan, M.J.; Lorenzo, A.V.: Cerebrospinal fluid perfusion studies in childhood hydrocephalus. Surg. Neurol. *1:* 317–320 (1973).

4 Standard Practice for Evaluating and Specifying Implantable Shunt Assemblies for Neurosurgical Application: Annual Book of ASTM Standards, part 46, F647, March 1980 (Am. National Standards Institute, New York 1980).

L.K. Page, MD, Professor and Chief of the Division of Pediatric Neurosurgery, University of Miami, Miami, FL 33101 (USA)

Monogr. neural Sci., vol. 8, pp. 199–201 (Karger, Basel 1982)

Diverse Clinical Applications of Percutaneous Lumboperitoneal Shunts

H.E. James[a], *P.B. Tibbs*[b]

[a]Division of Neurosurgery, Surgery, and the Department of Pediatrics University of California, San Diego, Calif.; [b]Division of Neurosurgery, Surgery, University of Kentucky Medical Center, Lexington, Ky., USA

Introduction

Cerebrospinal fluid (CSF) shunt procedures are frequently employed in clinical practice. The preferred shunts presently are ventriculoperitoneal and ventriculojugular-atrial. Peritoneal shunts are felt to require fewer revisions and have less severe complications. These shunts are mostly used for communicating and obstructive hydrocephalus. Lumboperitoneal shunts are less commonly employed. This is due to a combination of circumstances. For one, there must be evidence of communication between the spinal subarachnoid space and the intracranial space; also, previous reports refer to laminectomy as part of the procedure, and this has been felt to be one of the causes of subsequent scolioses developing in children [2]. The polyethylene tubing, previously employed, was felt by some authors to cause progressive arachnoiditis [1]. Those using lumboperitoneal shunts, however, refer to the simplicity of the placement of the shunt when compared to other cranial CSF shunts [3–5]. By the following we wish to present our clinical experience with lumboperitoneal shunts.

Materials and Methods

28 patients with ages ranging from 1 to 75 years were treated with lumboperitoneal shunts in this series. The population age range went from 1 to 75 years. There were 12 patients aged 19 years and under and 16 patients aged 20 years and over. The types of hydrocephalus or disease process for which they received the shunt are listed in table I. The 4 patients with cranial CSF fistulae acquired following surgery (3 transsphenoidal sellar procedures, 1 tuberculum meningioma), all of which had failed to seal with conservative measurements and CSF rhinorrhea persisted over 3 weeks. After no evidence of CSF infection was revealed by lumbar puncture, these patients were maintained on antibiotic coverage and a percutaneous lumboperitoneal shunt was inserted. There were 2 patients with recurrent

Table I. Type of hydrocephalus or disease process for which shunts were given

Diagnosis	Number of patients	
Communicating hydrocephalus	16	
Congenital		2
Newborn with hemorrhage		2
Following trauma		2
Following infection		3
Normal pressure		3
Adult subarachnoid hemorrhage		4
Pseudotumor cerebri	3	
Cranial CSF fistulae	4	
Postoperative sellar surgery		3
Traumatic		1
Spinal CSF fistulae (subcutaneous-peritoneal shunt)	3	
Bulging craniotomy site	2	

bulging of their craniotomy site. The primary diagnosis was head trauma in one and a brain tumor in the other. The bulging persisted over 4 weeks, with a CT scan indicating only minimal ventricular enlargement. A percutaneous lumboperitoneal shunt was then placed. 3 patients manifested recurring bulging and in one intermittent leakage of CSF in the lumbosacral region, following removal of a large leptomyelolipoma. These persisted for 2 or more weeks and created discomfort to the patients. A lumbar percutaneous subcutaneous-peritoneal shunt was then performed. The 3 patients with pseudotumor cerebri were females, and they were suffering from protracted headaches and visual difficulties despite intensive medical managements; on CT scan they demonstrated a very small ventricular system and no masses or displacements. Preoperative assessment varied in the group of patients with communicating hydrocephalus, according to the patient's age. In infants whose CT scan revealed ventricular enlargement which involved the fourth ventricles, a unilateral ventricle tap was performed and 0.5 ml of indigo carmine was exchanged for CSF. 1 h later lumbar puncture was performed, and if the CSF at that level was stained blue, communicating hydrocephalus was confirmed (Blackfan test). In older children and in adults in whom the clinical assessment and CT scan suggested communicating hydrocephalus, isotope cisternography was performed to document communication between the lumbar subarachnoid space and the ventricular system.

For the procedure, following endotracheal intubation and general anesthesia, the patients were placed in the right lateral decubitus position to expose the lumbosacral region and the left abdomen. A small incision was performed in the midline of the lumbar region and another in the left lower quadrant. A silk tie is then tunneled through both incisions, and a 14-gauge Touhey needle is employed for the lumbar puncture and for the insertion of the shunt tube into the subrarachnoid space. The needle is then withdrawn and the distal end of the shunt is tied with the previous tunneled silk tie; in this way the shunt tubing is passed to the abdominal incision. CSF should be flowing freely through the shunt once the silk tie is removed. The distal end is then inserted into the peritoneal cavity through a muscle-splitting procedure. We employ a barium-impregnated silastic single tube with an outer diameter of 0.065 cm, with lengths of 25, 50, or 80 cm (lumboperitoneal shunt tube, James design, Codman & Shurtleff, Inc., Randolph, Mass.). The tube has fenestrations for the subarachnoid space in its proximal portion and slits distally, as do most peritoneal shunts of ventriculoperitoneal tubing. This tube has a flow rate which ranges from 1 to 2 ml/min under hydrostatic column effect, with an opening pressure which ranges from 3 to 5.5 Torr.

Results

Of the 4 patients with cranial CSF fistulae that were treated, 3 ceased leaking following the shunt, and one failed to respond to the treatments requiring subsequently an operative procedure to occlude the leakage point. Of the 3 patients that had lumbar subcutaneous CSF fistulae, there was a successful response in all. In the 3 patients that had pseudotumor cerebri, there was a dramatic improvement in vision and headaches in all 3. Of the 2 patients with a bulging craniotomy site, 1 improved, and 1 subsequently went on to require a ventriculoperitoneal shunt for obstructive hydrocephalus. In the group with communicating hydrocephalus, there was an improvement noted with this treatment in 12 of the 13 patients over 4 months of age. However, all but 1 of 4 patients under 4 months failed to improve following the lumboperitoneal shunt. This was felt to be due to debris in the spinal fluid of infants with previous hemorrhage or infections. In the adult patients with the diagnosis of normal pressure hydrocephalus of idiopathic origin, there was an improvement clinically in 2 of the 3, with an interesting reduction of ventricles on follow-up CT scan only in 1 of these 2 patients. Of the adult patients treated with lumboperitoneal shunts following subarachnoid hemorrhage, there was clinical improvement in all 4. There was one shunt infection in the present series.

References

1 Hoffman, H.J.; Hendrick, E.B.; Humphreys, R.P.: New lumboperitoneal shunt for communicating hydrocephalus. Technical note. J. Neurosurg. *44:* 258–261 (1976).

2 Kushner, J.; Alexander, E., Jr.; Davis, C.H., Jr.; Kelly, D.L., Jr.: Kyphoscoliosis following lumbar subarachnoid shunts. J. Neurosurg. *34:* 783–791 (1971).

3 Murtagh, F.; Lehman, R.: Peritoneal shunts in hydrocephalus. J. Am. med. Ass. *202:* 1010–1014 (1967).

4 Scott, M.; Wycis, H.T.; Murtagh, F.; Reyes, V.: Observations on ventricular and lumbar peritoneal shunts in hydrocephalus in infants. J. Neurosurg. *12:* 165–175 (1955).

5 Spetzler, R.F.; Wilson, C.B.; Grollmus, J.M.: Percutaneous lumboperitoneal shunt. Technical note. J. Neurosurg. *43:* 770–773 (1975).

H.E. James, MD, Division of Neurosurgery, Surgery, and the Department of Pediatrics, University of California, San Diego, CA 92103 (USA)

Monogr. neural Sci., vol. 8, p. 202 (Karger, Basel 1982)

Indications and Results in Lumbar-Subarachnoid Peritoneal Shunting

C. Lapras, P. Bret, P. Carlioz

Service de Neuro-Chirurgie, Hôpital Neurologique, Lyon, France

The authors report their experience of lumbar-peritoneal shunting in 25 infants and children with communicating hydrocephalus. In one third of the cases, an aetiological factor is found, mainly subarachnoidal bleeding and also new-born meningitis. X-Ray findings show the communicating aspect of the hydrocephalus: during air encephalography, the contrast reaches enlarged lateral ventricles; CT scan studies with intrathecally injected metrizamide show the reflux of contrast into the ventricular system.

LP shunting was primarily performed in 10 cases and secondarily after aqueduct catheterism (3 cases) or after percutaneous ventriculostomy (1 case). In 9 cases, LP shunt was inserted after the failure of ventriculo-atrial shunt procedure and in 2 cases after the failure of both aqueduct catheterism and ventriculo-atrial shunting.

Results

(1) 1 patient died 3 months after surgery; fatal issue was not related to shunt dysfunction. (2) In most cases, postoperative course was uneventful. 1 patient required shunt revision. 1 patient developed bilateral inguinal hernia and another lumbar meningocele. No suppurative complication occurred. (3) Long-term follow-up shows: control of hydrocephalus is satisfactory with good psychomotor result in 12 cases; control of hydrocephalus with slight mental retardation in 4 cases; failure of hydrocephalus control requiring further surgical procedures in 7 cases. (4) 1 patient was lost to follow-up.

C. Lapras, MD, Service de Neuro-Chirurgie, Hôpital Neurologique, 59, Boulevard Pinel, F–69394 Lyon Cédex 3 (France)

Shunt Problems Related to the Etiology of Hydrocephalus

Monogr. neural Sci., vol. 8, pp. 203–205 (Karger, Basel 1982)

Introduction

C. Di Rocco

Istituto di Neurochirurgia, Roma, Italia

Despite its demonstrated effectiveness, enthusiasm with surgical treatment of hydrocephalus has been tempered by the recognition of a number of serious complications. In the case of the hydrocephalus accompanying congenital malformations of the central nervous system such a statement appears particularly true, as the well-known general complications of CSF shunts occur with distressing frequency, often assuming a life-threatening character.

Furthermore, surgical treatment of congenital maldevelopmental hydrocephalus is weighted by some peculiar complications, the importance of which should be stressed. Such complications derive from the complex interrelationship of the patient's primary disease, the development of compensatory mechanisms, and the type of treatment. Indeed, in maldevelopmental hydrocephalus, the proper selection of the patients and of the time of surgery might prove to be as important as the surgical procedure itself. In other words, complications and even mortality appear in many cases unquestionably related to errors in management and diagnosis.

In this direction, I would like to point out some particular situations, which express the above-mentioned complex interrelationship. The first – and maybe the easiest to be understood – is the condition where a severe congenital ventricular dilatation accompanies the almost complete absence of cerebral parenchyma. This can occur, for example, in cases of hydranencephaly and diffuse porencephaly. Different from what can be noticed in severe obstructive hydrocephalus where the CSF shunt insertion is followed, in most instances, by the cerebral cortex re-expansion, in this situation the drainage of fluid from the cranial cavity does not induce compensatory modifications in cerebral tissue volume. In this type of patient, we had a significant high incidence of complications, namely CSF fistulae around the ventricular catheter and inadequate low drainage and infections. A second condition, in which CSF shunting procedures show peculiar difficulties, is – on the contrary – harder to understand. I am referring to the cases in which the diversion of CSF is made possible by the presence of abnormal cavities, generally lying between the two cerebral hemispheres, in which the tip of the ventricular catheter is lodged. The communication between these cavities and the normal ventricular system cannot be appreciated on CT scan examination when the inserted CSF shunt assembly is functioning well.

For some aspects, namely the association with slit-like lateral ventricles, these children remind one of those patients described by *Hawkins et al.* [1], in whom the enlarged cavity was an isolated fourth ventricle. In all the children with this kind of anatomo-functional arrangement whom we encountered, a shunt dependency was present; clinical conditions deteriorated very fast when the CSF shunt ceased working. Attempts of obtaining a more suitable position of ventricular catheter failed in almost all instances.

In patients with congenital hydrocephalus compensatory mechanisms for CSF absorption develop early; in several cases they are so effective that an apparent or even real arrest of the syndrome may occur. A third situation, I would like to point out, concerns directly these compensatory processes. In older children, with slowly evolving ventricular dilatation or apparently arrested hydrocephalus the abrupt changes in the CSF dynamics, induced by the shunt insertion, often cause severe complications, such as, for instance, subdural hematomas. Changes in cerebrovascular compliance play a relevant role in these dangerous events. Consequently, the early correction of the hydrocephalus should be advocated: in fact it may prevent, at least in part, the secondary damage of cerebral parenchyma, which precociously takes place together with the development of alternative ways for CSF circulation and absorption, namely those associated with transependymal fluid migration.

Particularly interesting are those situations where the absorption mechanisms, even if defective, are still apt to hinder persistent states of intracranial hypertension. As suggested earlier in this symposium, the insertion of a CSF shunt may limit the ability to accommodate for an increase in the CSF pressure, so inducing an unwanted shunt dependency; this might be observed in patients with constrictive hydrocephalus when the shunt curtails the absorptive CSF mechanisms, acting at the high-pressure ranges. During the infusion test, these mechanisms are responsible for the decrease in intracranial pressure which takes place in the late phase of the examination. In some of these subjects, the factor causing the CSF dynamic disturbance may be corrected directly, as shown, for example, by the effectiveness of craniectomy in children with sagittal craniosynostosis.

The last situation that I would like to discuss is related to the possible decompensation of an abnormal, but stabilized, condition of intracranial pressure, which might be brought about by shunt surgery. The risks of such a complication were pointed out by *Raimondi* [2] when describing the upward herniation of cerebellar structures in the Dandy-Walker cyst following the decrease in supratentorial pressure. The same complication may occur in cases of posterior fossa arachnoid cyst, as we experienced once in a child with an arachnoid cyst located within the fourth ventricle, whose condition deteriorated after CSF shunting from the lateral ventricle. In fact, as stressed recently by *James et al.* [3], in the Dandy-Walker syndrome a posterior fossa mass effect may not respond to the lateral ventricle shunt assembly, so that a dual shunt placed from the ventricle and the posterior fossa cyst is advocated. This last example demonstrates in my opinion how, in the treatment of congenital hydrocephalus, the correct interpretation and the proper management of the syndrome might greatly contribute to reduce the incidence of complications which, consequently, do not depend entirely on the hydrocephalus itself.

References

1 Hawkins, J.C.; Hoffman, H.J.; Humphreys, R.P.: Isolated fourth ventricle as a complication of ventricular shunting. J. Neurosurg. *49:* 910–913 (1978).

2 Raimondi, A.J.; Samuelson G.; Yarzagary, L.; Norton, T.: Atresia of the foramina of Luschka and Magendie: the Dandy-Walker cyst. J. Neurosurg. *31:* 202–216 (1969).

3 James, H.E.; Kaiser, G.; Schut, L.; Bruce, D.A.: Problems of diagnosis and treatment in the Dandy-Walker syndrome. Child's Brain *5:* 24–30 (1979).

C. Di. Rocco, MD, Istituto di Neurochirurgia, Università Cattolica – Policlinico Gemelli, Largo Gemelli 8, I–00100 Roma (Italia)

Monogr. neural Sci., vol. 8, pp. 206–208 (Karger, Basel 1982)

Venous Obstruction in the Posterior Fossa as the Cause of Hydrocephalus

Mechanism of the Effects of Ventriculojugular Shunt

J. Andeweg

Provinciaal Ziekenhuis, Santpoort, The Netherlands

The current basic ideas about obstruction of cerebrospinal fluid (CSF) circulation as the cause of hydrocephalus were formed by *Dandy and Blackfan* [1914] and *Weed* [1922] in the two decades beginning 1914, and completed with articles by *Flexner* [1934] and by *Bedford* [1934a, b].

Flexner [1934] suggested that CSF is a secretion, because calculations based on the Donnan equilibrium (of *electrolytes* in plasma and CSF) would show that energy expenditure by the choroid plexus epithelium is required to produce CSF from plasma. The calculations of *Flexner* [1934] are not valid, however, because the (theoretical!) Donnan equilibrium is inexact. In the same way one might, therefore, have shown 'energy expenditure' even by a lifeless membrane in vitro. *Bedford* [1934a, b] suggested that occlusion of the great vein of Galen would not cause hydrocephalus. But he did his experiments on dogs and Rhesus monkeys; in these animals the basal veins terminate in the lateral sinuses, and a collateral pathway thus exists. In man the basal veins terminate in the great vein of Galen.

Neurology thus remained separated from the general physiology concerning cardiovascular system and tissue fluids. While daily CSF flow is estimated at 500 ml, it received (in regard to hydrocephalus and CSFP) more attention than the blood flow through the brain which amounts to more than 1,000 l a day. This large blood flow reflects the high cerebral metabolism: the adult brain consumes nearly 20% of the oxygen used by the body as a whole, and the newborn brain almost 50% [*Kety,* 1956]. Furthermore, the anatomy, physiology and pathology of cerebral *venous* flow were particularly neglected. About one million ml of blood has to leave the brain through the venous channels of the posterior fossa each day. This blood flows not only into the jugular veins, but also into the large vertebral vein system [*Batson,* 1957]. Also, venous drainage of the white matter and choroid plexuses occurs through the great vein of Galen, while the cerebral cortex is drained by the superficial cerebral veins [*Hédon,* 1888; *Ferner,* 1958a, b]. Because the great vein of Galen and the sigmoid sinuses are compressible end-channels, it is understandable that space-occupying processes will cause venous obstruction, especially when they are located in the posterior fossa. This will cause a rise of capillary pressure also in the choroid plexuses with their large surface. And thus CSFP will be elevated through the Starling *hydrostatic-osmotic pressure equilibrium* between CSF and plasma. Also, the increased venous resistance will reduce blood flow, and this in turn causes brain atrophy visible as enlargement of the ventricles (called hydrocephalus). When especially the deep venous system is obstructed, atrophy of the white matter will predominate as collateral flow to the superficial venous system is insufficient.

Experiments with postural change show that all pressures within the cardiovascular system have to be referred to a point of *constant* pressure (not exactly zero!) near the tricuspidal valves in the right heart [*Guyton and Greganti,* 1956]. Postural changes in CSFP can be related to this same point (at which the constant end-diastolic pressure is usually slightly negative). This illustrates the narrow relation between CSFP and venous pressures. Accordingly, right cardiac insufficiency causes a rise in CSFP.

According to *Welch and Friedman* [1960] the arachnoid villi are a one-way valve system from CSF space to dural sinus, governed only by difference in *hydrostatic* pressure. Intracranial venous obstruction will thus cause a rise in CSFP also through this mechanism. Direct connection between CSF space and jugular vein through a shunt (one-way valve) will circumvent intracranial venous obstruction and thus lower the CSFP. Lowering of the CSFP will cause a dilatation of subarachnoidal veins, resistance to blood flow will diminish accordingly and CBF will partially improve. The lowered CSFP exerts less pressure on the ependyma, and the brain will expand slightly because intracerebral fluid pressure remains elevated. Thus, the ventricles become smaller, a fact which was already mentioned by *Nulsen and Spitz* [1951] when they introduced the ventriculojugular shunt in 1951. The improvement in CBF will occur in the same way when a normal CSFP is lowered by ventriculojugular shunting [*Greitz et al.*, 1969; *Salmon and Timperman,* 1971]. As interstitial cerebral fluid increases, the cortical mantle becomes thicker, the ventricles accordingly become smaller, and the expanding midbrain may close the aqueduct after shunting.

Already many years ago several investigators disagreed with the findings and conclusions which *Dandy* presented in regard to experimental obstruction of CSF pathways [*Guleke,* 1930; *Hassin et al.,* 1937]. It should be added that *Dandy* never mentioned any CSFP measurement.

Explanation of hydrocephalus and intracranial hypertension by venous obstruction opens the way to the explanation of many clinico-pathological phenomena. Congenital hydrocephalus can thus be of *prenatal* origin (small posterior fossa due to hypoplasia of the chondrocranium causing Chiari hindbrain dislocation and compression of venous channels), or due to *birth injury* to venous channels of the posterior fossa and their constriction by dural fibrosis resulting from hemorrhage.

References

Batson, O.V. The vertebral vein system. Am. J. Roentg. *78:* 195–212 (1957).

Bedford, T.H.B.: The great vein of Galen and the syndrome of increased intracranial pressure. Brain *57:* 1–24 (1934a).

Bedford, T.H.B.: The venous system of the velum interpositum of the Rhesus monkey and the effect of experimental occlusion of the great vein of Galen. Brain *57:* 255–265 (1934b).

Dandy, W.E.; Blackfan, K.D.: Internal hydrocephalus. Am. J. Dis. Child. *8:* 406–482 (1914).

Ferner, H.: Die inneren Hirnvenen des Menschen und ihre Zustromgebiete. Verh. anat. Ges., *55:* 237–244 (1958a).

Ferner, H.: Anatomische und phlebographische Studien der inneren Hirnvenen des Menschen. Z. Anat. EntwGesch. *120:* 481–491 (1958b).

Flexner, L.B.: The chemistry and nature of the cerebrospinal fluid. Physiol. Rev. *14:* 161–187 (1934).

Greitz, T.V.B.; Grepe, A.O.L.; Kalmér, M.S.F.; Lopez, J.: Pre- and postoperative evaluation of cerebral blood flow in low-pressure hydrocephalus. J. Neurosurg. *31:* 644–651 (1969).

Guleke, N.: Über die Entstehung des Hydrocephalus internus. Arch. klin. Chir. *162:* 533–550 (1930).

Guyton, A.C.; Greganti, F.P.: A physiologic reference point for measuring circulatory pressures in the dog – particularly venous pressure. Am. J. Physiol. *185:* 137–141 (1956).

Hassin, G.B.; Oldberg, E.; Tinsley, M.: Changes in the brain in plexectomized dogs, with comments on the cerebrospinal fluid. Archs Neurol. Psychiat. Chicago *38:* 1224–1239 (1937).

Hédon, E.: Etude anatomique sur la circulation veineuse de l'encéphale (Paris 1888).

Kety, S.S.: Human cerebral blood flow and oxygen consumption as related to aging. J. chron. Dis. *3:* 478–486 (1956).

Nulsen, F.E.; Spitz, E.B.; Treatment of hydrocephalus by direct shunt from ventricle to jugular vein. Surg. Forum *1:* 399–403 (1951).

Salmon, J.H.; Timperman, A.L.: Effect of intracranial hypotension on cerebral blood flow. J. Neurol. Neurosurg. Psychiat. *34:* 687–692 (1971).

Weed, L.H.: The cerebrospinal fluid. Physiol. Rev. *2:* 171–203 (1922).

Welch, K.; Friedman, V.: The cerebrospinal fluid valves. Brain *83:* 454–469 (1960).

J. Andeweg, MD, Provinciaal Ziekenhuis, NL–2080 AB Santpoort (The Netherlands)

Monogr. neural Sci., vol. 8, pp. 209–212 (Karger, Basel 1982)

Non-Tumoral Hydrocephalus in Newborns

P. Frerebeau, M. Guillen, J.M. Privat, J. Benezech
Clinique Neuro-Chirurgicale, CHU, Montpellier, France

Neonatal hydrocephalus causes specific problems which belong to the progress of perinatality and only a few analytic series were published concerning this period exclusively. *Our series* comprises 39 cases of non-tumoral hydrocephalus, all operated during the first 3 months of life; the average postoperative course was 34 months with extreme values of 6 months and 7 years.

Concerning the *etiologies,* we found: Primitive malformative hydrocephalus: 36%, of which 78.5% were part of a polymalformative context. Acquired hydrocephalus: 64%, of which the larger part (80%) were consecutive to hemorrhagic (44%) or infectious (36%) processes. For the latter, *acquired risk factors* appear as specific to this population. Birth term (premature infants, 30%); birth weight (57% weighed less than 3 kg and 40% less than 2.5 kg) and neonatal complications (70% had an Apgar score less than 10 at the fifth minute of life). Other factors, such as primiparity (57%) and twin pregnancy (16%), also participate.

Treatment consisted of ventriculoperitoneal shunts (92.8%), ventriculoatrial shunts (4.2%) and percutaneous ventriculocisternotomies (2.8%). We performed 69 operations for the 39 patients of the series. The material used consisted essentially of low-resistance valves, of variable pressure according to preoperative ICP measures, with a majority of medium-pressure valves (56.9%).

Complications were frequent in a rather limited number of patients (40 complications in 13 patients) and were of two kinds: obstructive or infectious. We can note: (1) That *mechanical complications* at a so-called 'undetermined level' were frequent (12) but that 5 cases used low-pressure valves, which suggests the possibility of slit ventricles and that the other 7 cases shortly preceded an infectious complication, of which it seemed to be the initial manifestation. (2) Frequency and gravity of *infectious complications* by the newborn led us to observe strict precautions concerning asepsia before and during the operation and to draw systematic CSF samples from the material during the first 2 postoperative days with a short-term attempt to conserve the material by an early general and local antibiotic treatment in case of positive results.

Table I. Neonatal hydrocephalus. Prognostic factors at operation

	Results	
	GR (QD ⩾ 75)	BR (QD < 75)
Age		
0–15 days	1	2
15–30 days	3	1
30–90 days	17	3
Weight		
1,300–3,000 g	3	2
3,000 g	17	4

Results

Death rate: 30.6% (12 cases) which is subdivided into early mortality (6 cases) due to infections with a short delay (5 months) and dysfunctions with a longer delay (up to 5 years). By the survivals we find: 59.3% of 'good results': normal DPM according to age or QD ⩾ 100 ± minor character abnormalities without disturbance of integration. 18.5% of 'minor handicaps', that means slight disturbance or 75 < QD < 100 ± character abnormalities disturbing adaptation. 22.2% of 'major handicaps' with at the worst vegetative functions.

Discussion

Despite a great number of large series concerning long-term results after shunting procedures [2, 3, 5–7, 9], there is however a paucity of publications concerning the special aspects of hydrocephalus in the newborn [1, 4, 8, 10]. (1) It seemed to be interesting to consider that distinction between primitive and acquired hydrocephalus should be more difficult. In fact the study of *associated malformations* revealed their high frequency and that there exists no absolute concordance between these malformations and the primitive forms of hydrocephalus. (2) On the other hand results obtained were related to different factors which may or may not play a role in determining prognosis. In the first group we find *clinical factors* (table I).

Risky prognosis increases inversely according to age and weight at the time of the first operation: but there was, in this sort series, a non-significant variation according to etiology, initial clinical status and vital risk, as well as of

Table II. Operative technique

	Results		
	QD ⩾ 100	75 < QD < 100	QD < 75
Low pressure (n = 4) 5–30 mm H_2O	1	–	3
Medium pressure (n = 19) 45–80 mm H_2O	13	4	2
High pressure (n = 2) 95–125 mm H_2O	1	1	–
Percutaneous V° cisternostomy (n = 2)	2	–	–
Total (n = 27)	17	5	5

eventual ulterior complications and total duration of disease. In the second group we find *technical factors* (table II). Results related to kind of operation carried out show: that most of medium-pressure valves had led to good results, but that in 3 of 4 cases the low-pressure valves had led to major handicaps.

Conclusion

This study stresses three points: (1) The risk involved in too early operations of newborns with low weight, thus suggesting the necessity for transitory palliative treatment. (2) The necessity of early and rigorous discovery and treatment of infectious complications. (3) The importance of the choice of operative technique, which should consist, whenever possible, of internal shunting and if not of a careful choice of the pressure level of the valve. Progress in the preceding three areas will probably lead to a better long-term prognosis.

References

1 Bada, H.S.; Salmon, J.H.; Pearson, D.H.: Early surgical intervention in posthemorrhagic hydrocephalus. Child's Brain *5:* 109–115 (1979).
2 Descuns, P.; Lebatard-Sartre, R.; Collet, M.; Albrespy, C.: A propos de 74 cas d'hydrocéphalie non tumorale du nourrison opéré. Neuro-Chirurgie *17:* suppl. 5, pp. 71–77 (1971).
3 Forrest, D.M.; Cooper, D.G.W.: Complications of ventriculo-atrial shunts. A review of 455 cases. J. Neurosurg. *29:* 506–512 (1968).
4 Galibert, P.; Delcourt, J.; Grunewald, P.; Christiaens, J.L.: A propos de l'hydrocéphalie du prématuré: commun. SNCLF, Rennes 1967.
5 Guidetti, B.; Giuffre, R.; Palma, L.; Fontana, M.: Hydrocephalus in infancy and childhood. An experience of CSF shunting. Child's Brain *2:* 209–225 (1976).

6 Keucher, T.R.; Mealey, J.: Long-term results after ventriculo-atrial and ventriculo-peritoneal shunting for infantile hydrocephalus. J. Neurosurg. *50:* 179–186 (1979).
7 Lepoire, J.; Lapras, C.: Traitement de l'hydrocéphalic non tumorale du nourrisson par dérivation ventriculo-atriale. Neuro-Chirurgie *13:* 211–342 (1967).
8 Lorber, J.: Ventriculocardiac shunts in the first week of the life. Devl Med. Child Neurol. *20:* suppl., p. 13 (1969).
9 Mealey, J.; Gilmor, R.L.; Bubb, M.P.: The prognosis of hydrocephalus overt at birth. J. Neurosurg. *39:* 348–354 (1973).
10 Wise, B.L.; Ballard, R.: Hydrocephalus secondary to intracranial hemorrhage in premature infants. Child's Brain *2:* 231–241 (1976).

P. Frerebeau, MD, Clinique Neuro-Chirurgicale, CHU, F–34000 Montpellier (France)

Monogr. neural Sci., vol. 8, pp. 213–214 (Karger, Basel 1982)

Complications and Operative Procedure in Cases of Late Decompensated Huge Hydrocephalus

E. Markakis, G. Haensel-Friedrich, F. Theophilo, H. Vogelsang
Neurochirurgische Klinik, Hannover, FRG

The group of decompensated arrested hydrocephalus acquires a particular position within the large number of children with hydrocephalus from different origins, which after diagnosis required a valve system. These children reach a relatively advanced age without symptoms, in spite of a huge hydrocephalus without a shunt. They may develop either spontaneous progressive neurological signs and intracranial pressure symptoms or decompensate due to extracerebral noxa, for example cranial trauma or general infection.

5 children with arrested huge hydrocephalus between the ages of 2 and 10 years were treated in our clinic. 2 cases developed decompensation after a light cranial trauma. 2 others spontaneously developed neurological signs, such as tetraspastic, symptoms of intracranial hypertension, and pathological signs of the cranial nerves. The fifth child developed spontaneously an oculomotorius paresis which subsided after 2 months without treatment. A few weeks later the child suffered a light cranial trauma which resulted in decompensation with vomiting, unconsciousness, a right-sided oculomotorius paresis and a left-sided abducens paresis. All the symptoms disappeared after the shunt operation.

Because of the known risk of postoperative complications, such as subdural hygromas or subdural haematomas, we indicated the operation only after measuring the intracranial pressure. We recommend the epidural ICP measurement because with it we reduce the possibility of CSF problems, for example infection or CSF leakage after removal of ventrical catheter in cases of no indication for operation. In special cases we additionally implanted a ventrical catheter and measured the ventricle compliance. The ICP results in 3 of the 5 cases were over 50–60 mm Hg. In these cases we indicated operation because of high-pressure levels. The average pressure in 2 other cases was 15–20 mm Hg. We found, however, pathological plateau and B pressure waves or additional abnormal compliance.

Although we implanted a high-pressure shunt in all 5 cases, we observed 3 weeks postoperatively in 1 of our patients a complication in the form of a subdural hygroma with ventricle collapse. In another patient we observed a subdural haematoma due to tearing of a frontal bridge vein. The hygroma in the first case subsided 10 days after closing the shunt. In the second case we had to remove the left-sided haematoma by additional craniotomy.

In our opinion the indication for operation of late decompensated, until the time arrested, huge hydrocephalus should be considered only after ICP measurement and by evident neurological symptoms.

Postoperative complications appear usually until the 6th week. Complications in the form of relieving hygroma or subdural haematoma after these 6 weeks are unlikely. The children should be controlled within this period and computed tomography should be performed at the slightest suspicious clinical sign.

We implant a high-pressure shunt with an antisyphon device and an on-off system to check the valve's function and control postoperative complications. This way we can temporarily close the shunt without operation, should signs of ventricle collapse appear. We are considering the possibility of using the shunt only in a horizontal position (during the night) permitted by the on-off system, to eliminate hydrostatically induced over-functioning.

E. Markakis, MD, Neurochirurgische Klinik Hannover, D–3000 Hannover (FRG)

Monogr. neural Sci., vol. 8, pp. 215–217 (Karger, Basel 1982)

The So-Called Dandy-Walker Syndrome

Comments on Morphologic, Diagnostic and Therapeutic Problems

W. Entzian, B. Szepan, J. Wappenschmidt, F. Gullotta

Neurochirurgische Universitätsklinik,
Institut für Neuropathologie der Universität, Bonn, FRG

The Dandy-Walker syndrome needs a careful diagnostic and therapeutic approch, as it generally includes a space-occupying infratentorial cyst and an occlusive hydrocephalus. Our clinical and therapeutic experiences, which partially can be correlated with some new morphologic aspects, shall be demonstrated.

Patients

22 patients with the features of Dandy-Walker syndrome were observed and operated on in the period 1962–1979. 14 patients were admitted at an age of up to 12 months, 5 patients up to an age of 20 years, 3 patients up to an age of 30 years.

Clinical Diagnosis

Primary clinical symptoms of the babies were those of hydrocephalus, 1 baby additionally had an infratentorial meningocele. The children and adults however demonstrated cerebellar or brain stem symptoms, signs of raised intracranial pressure and hydrocephalic features in various combinations and degrees.

The final diagnosis of Dandy-Walker syndrome was achieved in pre-CT era only in half of the cases before the first therapeutical step, i.e. a ventriculo-atrial shunt of the accompanying hydrocephalus was performed. 1 shunted child even was observed as long as 15 years, until CT revealed the true diagnosis. Retrospectively, plain X-ray films, of the head of this boy, showed the progressive bulging of the posterior fossa.

Results of Therapy

In some patients only one operative procedure was performed, in others a two-step therapy had become necessary or was planned and carried out, as

Table I. Primary and secondary operations, performed in Dandy-Walker syndrome. Only 1 death is to be correlated to a postoperative complication, i.e. supratentorial decompressive hemorrhage after shunting of the cyst

Primary ventricular shunt		primary excision of cyst	
Only	8 (1 death)	only	3 (1 death)
Plus secondary excision of cyst	3 (1 death)	plus secondary	
Secondary combined shunt	2	ventricular shunt	1
Primary shunt of cyst		primary combined shunt (of ventricles and cyst)	
Only	1 (death)		
Secondary combined shunt	1	only	1
Secondary converted ventricular shunt	1		
Before operation	1(death)		

shown in table I. 2 of the 5 deaths were related to the Dandy-Walker syndrome: 1 baby died from intracranial hypertension before adequate decompressive therapy could be initiated. A 7-year-old girl, who was admitted with hydrocephalus and papilledema, died from supratentorial extracerebral decompressive hemorrhage after exploration and shunting of the Dandy-Walker cyst.

Morphologic Findings

The histological examination of the walls of the cyst revealed two types of membranes: Type A cysts have a wall consisting only of arachnoid and regular ependyma. Macroscopically these cysts appeared to be an extension of the 4th ventricle, which has a normal looking ependyma. Type B cysts have a wall with three constituents: between arachnoid and ependyma a layer of cerebellar tissue (cells of the molecular layer) are to be found. The entire membrane demonstrates all signs of fetal vascular destruction. Macroscopically these walls were thick and pale – at least the midline. The cysts were found to lie on the roof of the 4th ventricle. Roof and floor of the 4th ventricle in most cases were fused with each other causing an occlusive hydrocephalus. At least in one instance, however, the 4th ventricle was open anatomically, but was occluded functionally by the space-occupying cyst. CSF entered the cysts through one or more openings which were located in an area normally occupied by the aqueduct. We learned that these openings were not the aqueduct itself but rather secondary communicative openings between the aqueduct or the residual of the 4th ventricle and the cyst.

Correlation of Clinical and Morphological Findings

The dysontogenetic type A cysts were found in elder patients only (4, 25, 29 years). The clinical symptoms provided the indication for a primary posterior fossa approach and cystectomy.

The vascular type B cysts were found in patients, who generally needed either initial shunting of the accompanying hydrocephalus (4 cases, aged 4, 5, 6, 11 months) or excision of the cyst (1 case, 4 months). Beyond babyhood only 1 child, age 7 years, was admitted with this type of cyst.

Discussion

An infratentorial space-occupying cyst is generally described as a Dandy-Walker cyst. Morphologically, etiologically and – partially – clinically two types of cysts, located at an identical region should be held apart: The type A cyst – Dandy-Walker cyst sensu strictu – has all morphological signs of a malformation as described by Dandy and Blackfan. This type causes a relative late onset of clinical symptoms – mainly posterior fossa symptoms.

The space-occupying type B cysts, found between the cerebellar hemispheres and bordered by a relatively thick membrane, are encountered in babies and are the result of a vascular parenchymal destruction during fetal life. One may speak of a porencephaly of the vermis. The resulting occlusive hydrocephalus generally needs shunting as the initial measure. Excision of the cyst as a second procedure at a later age (pre-school time?) should be planned, or at least kept in mind.

W. Entzian, MD, Neurochirurgische Universitätsklinik, Institut für Neuropathologie der Universität Bonn, D–5300 Bonn 1 (FRG)

Monogr. neural Sci., vol. 8, pp. 218–219 (Karger, Basel 1982)

Shunt and Shunt Problems in Tuberculous Meningitis with Hydrocephalus

S.N. Bhagwati

Medical Research Center, Bombay Hospital, Bombay, India

Tuberculous meningitis is still common in India and some of the countries of South East Asia. It is often associated with impairment of cerebrospinal fluid (CSF) circulation that results in the occurrence of hydrocephalus. Hydrocephalus leads to raised intracranial pressure, a factor that adversely affects the course of the disease [1–3, 5]. Insertion of a shunt therefore becomes necessary in quite a few of these cases. As a result, hydrocephalus of tuberculous origin forms an important group of hydrocephalus of non-tumoural origin for which a shunt is inserted in our country.

Besides the usual problems one comes across with a shunt insertion, there are problems peculiar to the disease. Therefore, a study of 306 cases of tuberculous meningitis over a period of 12 years (1968–1978), 160 of whom needed a shunt insertion, was carried out and the following observations were made.

The commonest form of impairment of CSF circulation was a result of a block at the basal cisterns and cisterna ambiens by tuberculous exudate with communicating type of hydrocephalus in 129 cases. There was a fourth ventricular outlet block in 26 and aqueductal block in 5 cases. In 15 of these, there also existed an impairment of absorption of CSF by the arachnoid villi over the cortical surface.

Suwanvela [7] did report a case of tuberculous meningitis in which following ventriculoperitoneal shunt, the abdominal cavity was studded with tubercles. Should then one insert a shunt in a case of tuberculous meningitis when the disease is active? We had to insert a ventriculo-atrial shunt to relieve the raised intracranial pressure in many cases even though lumbar CSF showed an active disease. In none of these patients was there a miliary spread of the disease which one should have expected. This is probably due to the fact that though the lumbar CSF showed typical changes of tuberculous meningitis, ventricular CSF showed only marginal changes. Unless there is a tubercle on the choroid plexus or marked ependymitis, ventricular fluid tends to remain sterile. Also these children have been on vigorous antituberculous therapy for some time before surgery is undertaken and the same is continued for at least 1½ years. Hence shunt insertion in such cases does not lead to miliary spread of the disease.

The results of shunt insertion were very rewarding in cases in whom the sensorium was not much affected [2, 4]. In some of these patients who had some neurological deficit in the form of hemiparesis, dysphasia and visual impairment, a significant improvement occurred with regression of the neurological deficit after shunt insertion. The neurological deficit in such cases must have been a result of stretching of the arteries due to hydrocephalus with consequent ischaemia [6]. With the treatment of hydrocephalus, circulation in the ischaemic areas must have improved with regression of the neurological deficit. However, the results have been unsatisfactory in deeply stuporose, semicomatose and comatose patients. Of 48 such cases only 5 showed a complete recovery, 11 had residual hemiparesis with visual impairment, 5 remained in a vegetative condition and the rest died.

With these disheartening results, should a shunt be inserted or denied in such cases? As it has not been possible to determine the exact prognosticating factors in these cases, we do feel that a shunt be inserted in them even at the risk of having vegetative patients when there is a distinct hope of salvaging even a few of them.

Shunt dependency is usually present where the hydrocephalus is of an obstructive variety, as in the case of aqueductal stenosis or fourth ventricular outlet foramina block. In the case of the communicating variety, if the inflammatory exudate at the base of the brain gets resolved, the patient may become shunt-independent. However, if it is followed by fibrosis, impairment of CSF circulation persists and shunt remains a necessity. Shunt dependency is usually associated with all its attendant problems. Revision of the shunt had to be carried out once in 18 cases, twice in 3 and three times in 2 cases.

References

1 Bhagwati, S.N.; Singhal, B.S.: Raised intracranial pressure as a mode of presentation in tuberculous meningitis. Neurol. India *18:* 116 (1970).

2 Bhagwati, S.N.: Ventriculo-atrial shunt in tuberculous meningitis with hydrocephalus. J. Neurosurg. *35:* 309 (1971).

3 Bhagwati, S.N.; Singhal, B.S.: Raised intracranial pressure in tuberculous meningitis. Proc. 3rd Asian and Oceanian Congress of Neurology, 1971. Neurol. India *20:* suppl. 1, p. 80 (1972).

4 Bhagwati, S.N.; Singhal, B.S.: Ventriculo-atrial shunt in the treatment of tuberculous meningitis; in Kapila et al., Tuberculosis of the nervous system,

5 Dastur, D.K.; Lalitha, V.S.; Udani, P.M.; Paridh, U.: The brain and meninges in tuberculous meningitis – gross pathology in 100 cases and pathogenesis. Neurol. India *18:* 86 (1970).

6 Greitz, T.: Cerebral blood flow in occult hydrocephalus studied with angiography and the 133 xenon clearance method. Acta radiol. *8:* 376 (1969).

S.N. Bhagwati, MD, Medical Research Center, Bombay Hospital, Bombay (India)

Monogr. neural Sci., vol. 8, pp. 220–222 (Karger, Basel 1982)

Shunt Failure in Hydrocephalus with High-Protein Fluid

Emanuele Occhipinti, Carmine M. Carapella
Department of Neurosurgery, Istituto Regina Elena, Roma, Italy

Shunt failure in a series of 10 cases of hydrocephalus with high-protein fluid is examined. The follow-up was complicated in every case by malfunction of the shunt which required repeated revisions. The aetiology of this kind of hydrocephalus is discussed and the value of shunting procedures in such cases is critically reviewed.

We should like to summarize our experience in treating hydrocephalic children who have high-protein fluid. Out of a series of 155 cases we selected 10 cases where the protein content exceeded 1g/1.000 ml (table I). Aetiologically these cases were as follows: 6 cases of congenital hydrocephalus including one with diffuse melanosis; 2 cases of postmyelomeningocele hydrocephalus and ventriculitis, and 2 cases of posthaemorrhagic hydrocephalus, with cisternal blockage (table II).

Diagnosis was ascertained by CT scan or air ventriculography. In all cases a CSF shunt was performed, using a Pudenz or Holter valve system; 4 ventriculo-atrial (VA) and 6 ventriculoperitoneal (VP) shunts. All cases had to be revised. In 9 cases multiple revisions were necessary because of the obstruction of the ventricular catheter. In 2 cases with VP shunt a VA conversion was needed due to peritoneal malabsorption.

In 1 case (No. 2), at the fourth revision it was decided to insert a valveless shunt, consisting of a simple VP catheter. The immediate result was amazing, with dramatic resolution of the increased intracranial pressure and reduction of the head circumference. But after 2 months the child was again admitted to our department with a recurrence of increased intracranial pressure. To our surprise, an X-ray examination showed that the whole catheter had migrated into the right lateral ventricle, an unusual complication already mentioned in literature. In 3 other cases an extra-low pressure shunt was inserted.

The final result was unsatisfactory in all but 2 cases. Furthermore, in 3 cases (No. 2, 6, 9) the repeated revisions had caused ventriculitis, which created further

Table I. CSF protein content in a series of 10 cases of hydrocephalus

Cases	Sex	Age	CSF pre-operative protein content, mg/1,000 ml
1	M	7 days	2,500
2	F	2 months	4,500
3	M	1 month	1,900
4	F	20 days	1,930
5	F	6 months	1,050
6	F	4 days	3,100
7	F	20 days	1,850
8	M	2 months	1,100
9	F	25 days	2,300
10	M	6 months	2,100

Table II. Aetiology of 10 cases of hydrocephalus with high-protein fluid

Aetiology	Cases
Congenital hydrocephalus (1 case with diffuse melanosis)	6
Postmyelomeningocele hydrocephalus and ventriculitis	2
Tetraventricular posthaemorrhagic hydrocephalus with cisternal blockage	2

complication, because there were now both CSF pleocytosis and high-protein content. 5 died, 3 have severe impairment of psychomotor development, and 2 are in reasonable condition with an extra-low pressure shunt. In the light of this negative experience, what should be done in cases with high-protein fluid?

At the beginning external drainage may be advisable while waiting for the protein level to fall and evaluating CSF production rate. However, we have found this to be of little use. If therefore seems better to insert an extra-low pressure shunt at the beginning even at the risk of over-shunting. A peritoneal shunt is preferable because one can then, if really necessary, use a valveless system. Nevertheless, we have observed 2 cases of peritoneal malabsorption. One should also be more selective, and right from the start exclude from the treatment those cases of congenital hydrocephalus with serious malformations and high-protein fluid.

A problem yet to be solved is whether the shunt failure in these cases is due only to physical changes in the CSF, increased viscosity, changes in the flow inside rigid tubes, and to chemical changes in CSF protein present in pathological amounts, or is there an unknown factor which is responsible for the precipitation of protein, and consequent blockage of the valve system? We have recently begun to study this, together with our clinical analysis laboratory, but are not yet able to offer any information. If we could isolate a causative factor, we might be able to do more to help these children who have not only hydrocephalus, but hydrocephalus with high-protein fluid.

E. Occhipinti, MD, Department of Neurosurgery, Istituto Regina Elena,
Viale Regina Elena, 291, I–00161 Roma (Italy)

Monogr. neural Sci., vol. 8, pp. 223– 226 (Karger, Basel 1982)

Establishing the Diagnosis of Shunt Independence

Harold L. Rekate, Frank E. Nulsen, Harriet L. Mack, Glenn Morrison
Division of Neurosurgery, University Hospital of Cleveland, Cleveland, Ohio, USA

Despite careful programming of shunt revision to preserve function with a large population of hydrocephalic children, the clinician is occasionally faced with a shunt that has ceased to function in a totally asymptomatic patient. This serendipitous finding leads to the certain conclusion that not all patients once shunted require shunts for life. This study deals with the 36 patients out of a total hydrocephalic patient population of 271 who have been proven to be shunt-independent and the 17 patients who were unable to tolerate trial shunt occlusion.

Patient Selection

271 children with hydrocephalus of various etiologies are presently being followed at the Hydrocephalus-Myelodysplasia Clinic at the University Hospitals of Cleveland and form the basic study group for this analysis. 2 patients who have died within the past 10 years will also be discussed.

Results

In 51 of these patients need for elective shunt revision or the finding of a disconnected or too-short catheter led to a trial of shunt occlusion, either by ligation in the earlier phases of this study or more recently by the placement of an on-off valve. In 36 of these patients either with congenital communicating hydrocephalus (24 cases) or the Arnold-Chiari malformation (12 cases) occlusion was successful. Each of these children has been followed for at least 1 year with follow-up psychometric evaluation and measurement of ventricular size either through ventriculography or computerized tomographic (CT) scanning. In none of these patients has there been any evidence of intellectual, emotional or motor deterioration and the cerebral mantle has stabilized. We have not been successful in proving shunt independence in a single patient with non-communicating hydrocephalus and have abandoned the enterprise.

In 17 patients trial shunt occlusion (15) and removal (2) resulted in an unacceptable clinical situation. 5 patients suffered crises of intracranial hypertension 12 h to 5 years following shunt occlusion or removal resulting in 2 deaths and intellectual (2 patients) and motor and intellectual deterioration in the other 3. 1 patient began life with communicating hydrocephalus, but was converted to non-communicating following a *Streptococcus viridans* meningitis. She became comatose with bilateral decerebrate rigidity 12 h following shunt occlusion with an on-off valve. The shunt was reconstituted promptly, but the Parinaud's syndrome resolved slowly and she is left with a severe deficit in recent memory. The other 4 patients all had the Arnold-Chiari malformation with high level (thoraco-lumbar) meningomyeloceles. 1 patient died suddenly at home 9 months after shunt removal. A second patient suffered a respiratory arrest 12 h following shunt occlusion. He remained respirator-dependent for his remaining 7 months of life. The remaining 2 patients suffered respiratory arrests 3 days and 5 years after shunt occlusion, leading to severe neurologic downgrading.

There have been no serious complications from the trial occlusion of shunts in children with communicating hydrocephalus and we have been successful in 80% of the children whom we have attempted to challenge or 25% of the total population of children with communicating hydrocephalus. In 3 of these patients the experiment was abandoned with reluctance due to the subtleness of the complaints. In 1, a removed shunt was reinserted after the patient complained of morning headaches and blurred vision 6 weeks after its removal. In 2 others, mild symptoms of anorexia and mild listlessness were evaluated using a telemetered intracranial pressure monitoring device. These tracings revealed the appearance of plateau waves during sleep and resting high pulse pressure with normal intraventricular pressure. It was felt that both of these patients still had an active hydrocephalic process and their shunts were restored.

Intelligence Testing

Children with hydrocephalus are followed at regular intervals with psychometric testing beginning with Denver developmental testing in the first 3 years of life. Following this the child receives Stanford Binet or Wechsler intelligence scale for children (Wisc) tests. 15 of the 36 patients proven to be shunt-independent have had serial psychometrics available for analysis before and after the shunt occlusion or removal. There is a great deal of variation from year to year in these children with or without any hardware manipulation. There was no significant difference in the pre- and postocclusion full scale intelligence quotients either individually or as a group with only one exception, a patient whose IQ rose from 93 to 116 in a slowly progressive manner over 6 years following shunt occlusion. No evidence can be found in this group for the concept of insidious intellectual downgrading in the clinical asymptomatic patient.

Discussion

Foltz [3] stated that in 180 patients he had seen only 1 patient who was able to eventually do without the shunt and concluded 'once a shunt always a shunt'. *Nulsen and Becker* [5] stated that the development of later shunt independence was not only desirable but very possible. *Young et al.* [6] have shown that a normal sized ventricular system is not a requisite for adequacy of shunting or normal intellectual development and felt that a 3.5 cm mantle should be the goal of treatment of hydrocephalus by whatever techniques.

Numerous articles have been published since the Workshop in Hydrocephalus initiated the debate [3, 5]. Views range from that of *Foltz* [3] to *Holtzer and De Lange* [4] who feel that a substantial number of patients previously shunted may become shunt-independent at a later time regardless of ventricular size or etiology of hydrocephalus. Other authors feel that the diagnosis of shunt independence or shunt-independent arrest of hydrocephalus should only be made with extreme caution [1, 2].

The findings in the present study support the concept that the diagnosis of shunt independence must be made with care, but refute the concept that all children once shunted will require their shunt for life. Some conclusions seem justified from the data presented. Patients with non-communicating hydrocephalus are extremely unlikely to develop shunt independence without extreme ventriculomegaly and increased intracranial pressure leading to increase in transependymal absorption. This is not acceptable and we consider all children with non-communicating hydrocephalus shunt-dependent for life. Quite the reverse situation is true in the case of communicating hydrocephalus. Especially, but not exclusively, when the hydrocephalus begins after the perinatal period the chance of eventual shunt independence is quite good. Insidious, asymptomatic intellectual deterioration does not seem to occur and the child is obviously ill if shunt occlusion is not going to be tolerated.

In children with the Arnold-Chiari malformation and communicating hydrocephalus, the situation is quite different. 12 of these children have tolerated their shunt occlusions without difficulty. 4 others however suffered crises from their shunt occlusions and these occurred quite insidiously in 2 of these as late as 5 years later. These children seem to be inordinately at risk for difficulty. Possibly this would be due to the anatomic relationships at the cervicomedullary junction.

It is conceivable that suboccipital decompression prior to shunt occlusion might ameliorate the risk but this is purely theoretical.

Conclusion

Shunt independence is an obtainable and worthwhile goal in children with communicating hydrocephalus. Trial occlusion does not lead to asymptomatic intellectual deterioration but to definite symptoms in patients who do not tolerate this occlusion. Children with non-communicating hydrocephalus are unlikely to become shunt-independent. The risks of late decompensation in children with the Arnold-Chiari malformation demand the recommendation that these patients be considered shunt-dependent for life once this shunt is placed at all.

References

1 Blesser, M.; Coltheart, G.; Johnston, I.; Wright, J.: Intracranial pressure changes in 'arrested' hydrocephalus; in Shulman et al., Intracranial pressure IV, pp. 492–493 (Springer, Berlin 1980).

2 Di Rocco, C.; Caldarelli, M.; Maira, G.; Rossi, G.: The study of cerebrospinal fluid dynamics in apparently 'arrested' hydrocephalus in children. Child's Brain *3:* 359–374 (1977).

3 Foltz, E.: The first seven years of a hydrocephalus project; in Shulman, Workshop in hydrocephalus, pp. 79–114 (Children's Hospital of Philadelphia, Philadelphia 1965).

4 Holtzer, G.; De Lange, S.: Shunt independent arrest of hydrocephalus. J. Neurosurg. *39:* 698–701 (1973).

5 Nulsen, F.; Becker, D.: The control of progressive hydrocephalus in infancy by valve-regulated venous shunt; in Shulman, Workshop in hydrocephalus, pp. 115–150 (Children's Hospital of Philadelphia, Philadelphia 1965).

6 Young, H.; Nulsen, F.; Weiss, M.; Thomas, P.: The relationship of intelligence and cerebral mantle in treated infantile hydrocephalus. Pediactrics, Springfield *52:* 38–44 (1973).

H.L. Rekate, MD, Division of Neurosurgery, University Hospitals of Cleveland, Cleveland, OH 44106 (USA)

Monogr. neural Sci., vol. 8, pp. 227–228 (Karger, Basel 1982)

Can a Shunt Be Removed?

R. Hemmer

Neurosurgery Department of the University of Freiburg, Freiburg, FRG

The simplest justification to remove a shunt is the fact of a non-functioning of the drainage system over several weeks or months without any clinical signs of increased intracranial pressure. The shunt can be removed provided that the disturbed function is verified by X-ray (e.g. disconnection of the system, calcifications, percutaneous cannulization of the valve or flushing device with injection of contrast medium and confirming of the blockage). Continuous measurement or often repeated measurement of the ventricular pressure may be necessary to confirm the indication. Without doubt the ventricular pressure has to be checked before removal.

Over a period of 15 years we could remove the shunt in 40 of 444 children, i.e. in 9%. The exact data are: in hydrocephalus communicans 26 removals (9%) with 17 times compensation (65%), in myeloceles 14 removals all with full compensation. Moreover, the shunt could be removed in 4% during operation in cases where a preventive new implantation was intended. The follow-up studies showed no deterioration in school performance or mental development.

It is remarkable that one third of the children with communicating hydrocephalus need a new shunt after months or years. We excluded from our removals cases with obstructive hydrocephalus. It seemed to us too dangerous because there is only little breadth of compensation.

After shunt removal the children must be controlled very carefully. The decompensation may be announced only by intermittent headaches without clinical signs of increased pressure and without increasing of ventricular dilatation in the computer tomography. Generally the children who had a shunt removal in compensated hydrocephalus show a ventricular dilatation of different grades in the CT controls 7–19 years after the removal. The maximal hydrocephalus had an IQ within the normal limit (fig. 1).

The percentage of shunt removals is very low. It is recruited from those cases which have a tendency to compensate and which induced Lorber and

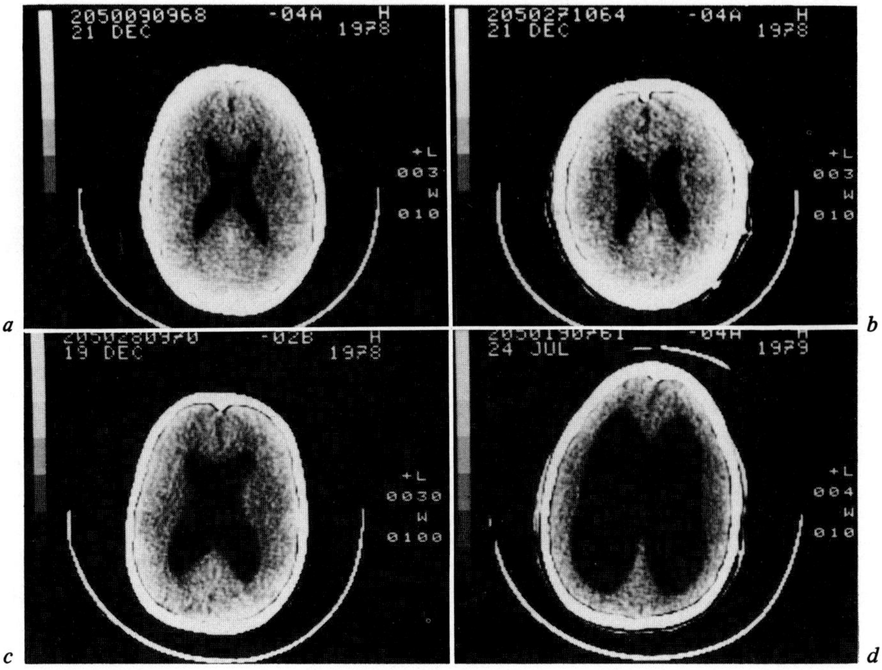

Fig. 1. Different grades in the CT controls 7–19 years after shunt removal: IQ = 106 (*a*), 110 (*b*), 129 (*c*), 111 (*d*).

Epstein-Ransohoff to treat conservatively. In my opinion the risk of brain damage with conservative treatment is too high and we do not have prior to a shunt operation any possibility to assert whether the hydrocephalus might compensate spontaneously.

As pointed out in 1976 [1] the removal of the drainage system without sufficient indication is a serious risk which often leads to emergency situations. For a greater part of the shunted children the saying is valid: 'Once a shunt – always a shunt.'

Reference

1 Hemmer, R.; Böhm, B.: Once a shunt, always a shunt? Devl Med. Child Neur. *18:* suppl. 37, pp. 69–73 (1976).

R. Hemmer, MD, Neurosurgery Department of the University of Freiburg,
D–7800 Freiburg (FRG)